The Kortum Technique

The Kortum Technique

How to Access the Human Body's Natural
Blueprint for Health and Healing

By
John Christopher Kortum

To order additional copies of this book, contact:
Xlibris
1-888-795-4274
www.Xlibris.com
Orders@Xlibris.com
60910

CONTENTS

To all children and to those who once were, may you

explore your senses with boundless unity

"Your ability to perceive indicators depends on how deeply you are willing to renew your discovery of the senses."

—*JCK*

FOREWORD

I MET JOHN Kortum for the very first time several years ago as I was seeing patients in my medical office in Bethesda, Maryland. He had contacted Dr. Len Wisneski, an associate of mine, about a new physical assessment technique he had developed that involved the use of *visual health indicators (organ indicators)*. Len and I were both intrigued and immediately full of questions regarding the efficacy of John's visual health indicators and the science behind it.

John described the identification of the organ indicators as part of his personal voyage of discovery. Since childhood, he had noticed distinct visual patterns and features in people's faces and bodies. Over the course of many years, he began to recognize these patterns as visual clues to illness. He learned to decode the symbols and developed an entire symbology and health assessment lexicon that was able to identify organ dysfunction without expensive laboratory testing! We asked if he would be able to demonstrate by *reading* the health issues of willing patients in our practice. He agreed, and it turned out that he was correct in every circumstance. We wondered how his technique would fare when tested within the rigors of a formal research process. We later designed and implemented a proof-of-concept study with positive results.

As we delved deeper into our work with John's technique, I was reminded of observations that I had made over the years in my work as a hospital nurse and integrative nurse practitioner. I too noticed that certain illnesses seemed to carry with them subtle visual characteristics. Although I could not describe them in concrete terms, I observed that smokers on the respiratory wards, heart-attack patients, and others seemed to look different from healthier individuals. At the time, I thought my observations were inconsequential. I now see that I was observing the visual health indicators of my patients and that these characteristics can be of tremendous use and value in evidence-based medicine and beyond. Further considering John's experience and my own in hindsight, I wondered whether others might be able to learn this technique; that is the subject of this book.

The Kortum Technique is an intuitive yet accessible (in the sense that it is a technique that can be learned) tool that provides the practitioner access to encoded information that is stored in the body and mind. As such, trained individuals may use it to recognize health and illness characteristics that relate to specific organ systems. It may also offer clues that lead to early diagnosis and treatment of significant health problems such as heart disease or cancer.

Furthermore, the Kortum Technique transcends medical diagnosis as we know it. The discovery of health indicators has the potential to support, enrich, and propel our journey of the soul forward. It gives those with the patience to learn it an interactive medium for understanding and interacting with their physical and nonphysical self. In time, this interaction develops into a deep and abiding relationship that holds clues to health, disease, and vitality. In fact, it shows us healing in a new paradigm as a nonlinear process that is accessible only through the recognition, communication, and affirmation of the nonphysical self. It offers a deeper, wiser, and more meaningful experience of healing to our clients and ourselves. As we forge deeper and deeper into these relationships that represent this inner source of healing, we move to the forefront of spirit-based integral medicine, the medicine of our future.

This book presents the theoretical framework and concepts that form the foundation for the Kortum Technique. It will help you to answer some fundamental questions such as

- What is the Kortum Technique?
- How does the Kortum Technique work?
- What differentiates the Kortum Technique from other forms of medical intuitive perception?
- How can I use this technique as an adjunct to my practice?

Some further questions for you to consider as you read are

- What is the organ that does the perceiving?
- Does it have a structure?
- How can the technique be used to empower people on their journey toward health and vitality?

Beyond the Kortum Technique itself, my work with John has helped me to remember that an open, questioning, and discriminating mind has an incredible potential for discovery. Recall, if you will, the many times in history when this has been so. When much of the civilized world thought that the world was flat, the great explorers, Marco Polo, Christopher Columbus, and others, ventured out beyond the horizon without missing a step. The many inventors who dared to think beyond ordinary parameters produced the cotton gin, the telegraph, and the electric light bulb. And in the scientific realm of medicine, a century ago, Wilhelm Conrad Roentgen and Marie Curie discovered and cultivated the use of X-rays, which enabled us to see for the first time inside a living, breathing individual; its implications were far reaching.

These major advances represented the mere discovery of *previously unrecognized* scientific phenomena. In essence, a change in perspective enabled us to see something previously undetectable. So too does the existence of healthy and diseased energies (indicators), and our ability to recognize them, embrace heretofore unrecognized territory, to wit, something previously undetectable that serves to challenge not only our methods of perceiving health and disease but also its relationship to the human condition. The assessment technique allows us to identify specific signs of illness and offers us an opportunity to reconsider the very nature of health itself. As you learn to recognize the visible energetic markers (indicators) of health (visible if you know where to look) you become part of a movement to forge a new frontier in health that is grounded not only within the physical boundaries of the body but beyond them as well. The evolution of this new outlook on wellness integrates and embraces all of the depth and complexity that is the human organism.

By cultivating a mere change in perspective, culled with an open and questioning mind, I have not only developed a powerful new tool for my practice but also a way of approaching health and wellness that is transpersonal—well beyond the everyday confines of a problem oriented medical system. As such, the integrative roots of disease can be exposed, thus creating fertile ground for true cure. My goal as a health care provider has always been to discover the bottom line concerning health and disease. Working at the level of the subtle distinctions that are required to recognize health indicators has helped me to lift some of the limiting borders of preconceived expectations and narrow definitions that constrain thinking. Getting outside the proverbial box has opened for me new worlds of thought and experience.

As you journey forward on your own introduction to the Kortum Technique, it will be important to remember to keep that open, questioning, and discriminating mind, being aware of the subtle distinctions that are available to be shifted and perceived in order to make room for that brave new world in each of us. As engineer and inventor Charles F. Kettering, (1876-1958) once said, "There exist limitless opportunities in every industry. Where there is an open mind, there will always be a frontier."

Beth H. Renné, MSN, ANP-C
Integrative Nurse Practitioner
Gestalt Therapist
Mind-Body Specialist
August 2009

PREFACE

A N ADVENTURE AWAITS the reader of this book: one that contains discovery, self-actualization, and innovation. It is a story that details the development of the Kortum Technique or Visual Assessment Process. This process has great potential to serve and support our health care system and its consumers. I first became aware of it several years ago when John approached me with the desire to demonstrate this method that he had been cultivating over a period of thirty years. The Kortum Technique is the result of his lifelong work.

As I considered his request and the possibility that it could ultimately be of benefit to my patients, I remembered how many of my colleagues had questioned me when I decided to study acupuncture and incorporate it into my medical practice. My reasoning at the time was quite simple: a scientifically oriented physician should learn and study techniques and modalities which have the ability to support the health and well-being of his or her patients.

When John explained that he was able to study a person, read health indicators, and formulate an assessment, I was intrigued and wondered if science would support his claims. To this end, we designed a pilot study to explore how the technique worked. We used the Integrative Internal Medicine practice in Bethesda, Maryland, that Beth Renné and I had developed as a test location and subject pool.

The book describes how Beth assisted with the scientific documentation and coached John to crystallize his gift into a coherent system which could be documented, understood, and taught to others. Although our study included only forty-five patients, our results demonstrated an accuracy of approximately 90 percent.

Throughout the process of the study, we discovered that an important side benefit of the technique is the gift of teaching others to see the world in a refreshing new way that is perhaps reminiscent of the freshly awakened senses we command as children.

The fact that the Kortum Technique can be taught to consumers as well as health care professionals is of great importance especially in this time of flux in our health care system. It is easy to envision this Visual Assessment Process as a cost-effective method for observing health imbalances as well as aid in diagnosis and treatment, when employed in conjunction with a licensed health care provider.

Finally, it is important to note, as mentioned previously, that this book is about self-actualization. John's story is a lesson for all of us. It is a courageous account of one man's passage as he learns to appreciate his innate gifts, even if they are not understood by the surrounding culture, and his quest, to follow his calling to serve humanity.

Enjoy the book as I have. Reading it is a fascinating journey.

Leonard A. Wisneski, MD, FACP
Clinical Professor of Medicine
George Washington University Medical Center

Adjunct Professor of Physiology & Biophysics
Georgetown University School of Medicine

ACKNOWLEDGMENTS

THE DEVELOPMENT OF the Kortum Technique became possible because of the opulent vision and full mettle of Leonard A. Wisneski and Beth H. Renné. Their devotion to imbue the perimeter of medical tradition, and explore the deep interiors of the human body, heart, mind, and spirit is an illuminating example for all health care professionals to follow.

Equally important and essential to the success of our research were all the patients who participated in the clinical study. The willingness of these courageous people to partake in such uncommon research has allowed the human body's language of health to come forth with medical substance.

I am eternally grateful to Beth for her assistance, guidance, wisdom and many hours of dedication in the organization of this manuscript. In addition, I would like to thank Beth's husband Mark and their two sons, Josh and Ben, for allowing her to be away from home in order to conduct our research and for the many times their kitchen table turned into an editorial caucus. Also, thanks to Beth's brother, Dave, by experimenting with our techniques, and giving us feedback about their reliability, we learned that healthy skepticism can also awaken the natural powers of perception.

I express my loving gratitude as a son to my mother and father for providing me with the ideal childhood environment that evoked this path of discovery. May both of you now find comfort in those turbulent days of my youth, knowing that it was nothing more than my frustration from *trying* to fit a multifaceted sensory peg into the round hole of the everyday world.

My sincere appreciation to Virginia Penny Holmes, for her elucidating perceptivities during all our conversations about life, great and small, in the control room at The Monroe Institute—*Lumos Maxima!*

Special thanks to those who supported me through the challenges that anyone encounters when bringing forward a new order of information. To Sue Wolfe, for her endless therapeutic telephone availability during the most interesting of times. To Cliff Young, for the true alliance of a friend and colleague and sharing his expertise. To Wayne Byars and Jean-Louis Falck, for their generous companionship and encouraging counsel near the Seine. To Shaye Hudson, for his comical camaraderie and brilliant wit. To Anne Legge, for showing me the success to writing is rewriting and tenacity. To Barbara Bowen, for explaining the ways and means of the publishing process, and listening with a truly patient ear. To the healing hands and heart of Debbie Grainger, for being a phenomenal massage therapist and confidante. To Cindy Kilduff, for her bright spirit and eternal laugh. To Liz Keehan-Kirby, for reminding me to look for miracles every day and to Madeleine L'Engle, for all the *Wrinkles*.

Most of all, my deepest gratitude is to Eiko—whose beautiful ribbon of love, reaches around the world from Tokyo to Paris to New York to Washington, DC, to my heart. Her unconditional support, keen insights, and deeply caring ways fill me with enchantment and affection. Our unity has transformed me into the man I have always aspired to be.

INTRODUCTION

WE ARE ALL on a subconscious pilgrimage, each one of us pursuing our individual path of life embedded with symbols and signs along the way. Mine tenuously emerged as a boy. While playing in abandoned nineteenth-century houses, I became filled with the undeniable urge to look for secret passages. A day at the quarry became my private archeological dig, convinced that the translation stone of an ancient language lay beneath my feet. Tales of hidden jewels in castles intrigued me beyond measure. My curiosities driven to a concealed world of significance but fueled by reasons I could not explain.

Just when my journey seemed completely without note, clues would surface to guide the way. The clues were subtle, seldom apparent, and oftentimes required interpretation. As I grew, all I knew was that I was supposed to find *something*.

I interpreted my childhood experiences to mean that ventures abroad and treasure troves were my destination. When I came of age, I moved easily into a career that required extensive travel; however, *something* was always missing. My worldly travels evoked questions, and anything that did not fit into our ordinary box of reality fascinated me. Slowly, the metaphor of my global pursuits manifested; and my destiny was not faraway lands and distant shores, as I had expected. Instead, my search turned my vessel to the topography of my *inner* landscape, a journey to the center of human sensory perception.

I navigated my mind through the deep waters of awareness and sailed the unfamiliar latitudes of thought. I spent years at sea, watching and waiting, when one day I made a peculiar discovery. Below the decks of intellect and behind the freight of logic and reason, I found a pelorus of the senses. It was there that I learned to see the unseen, feel the unfelt, hear the unheard, and I recovered the human body's natural maps for health and healing hidden in the faces of the people you see every day.

At the dawn of the twenty-first century, the realm of the five senses and human perception remains largely uncharted. Our current perspective of reality represents only a fraction of knowledge in our evolutionary progress along a frontier of infinity. When it comes to understanding human health, we live with the well-established reality that the human body *is* a certain way. A popular trend to understanding this notion is scientifically based. The general premise is the human being is a living chemistry set and that we can influence our chemical composition, and subsequently our health, by the aversion of toxins and the addition of nutrients or pharmaceutical products, fitness and exercise.

Another popular trend is the mind, body, and spirit connection. The general premise is there are ethereal bonds between the body chemistry and the mental, emotional, and spiritual forces of the human being. Again, the notion is that we can influence the chemical composition and subsequently our health through meditation, psycho or organic therapies, and positive thinking.

There is evidence and truth in either of these trends, but could there be more going on than meets *just* the eye?

What if the human being is more accurately described as an *alchemistry* set? What if as we affect our quality of health and well-being through health care and the transmutation of limiting thoughts and beliefs, our biological stake creates a metamorphosis of healing that can actually be observed by traits generated from the human body that are visible to the naked eye?

Furthermore, if every human being is biologically equipped with these observable traits, then it stands to reason that every human being is biologically equipped with the sensory hardware necessary to perceive these observable traits. This information suggests that there is considerably more to the human species than previously recognized.

The notion that the human body projects an encoded reference of health information that can be detected by simply looking at a person sends waves through the still waters of conventional thought. New paradigms can often be uncomfortable because it requires us to re-examine the reality we so preciously embrace. It is often easier to cling to traditional beliefs than accept the possibility that our version of reality may not be accurate or that we do not know as much as we thought.

However, new paradigms can also be exciting, especially if they cause us to refresh the reality we perceive. Human perception is highly subjective, and each one of us sees the world in our own unique way. Had these perceptions of the body's traits been uniquely my own I would have kept them to myself. However, since the people I have taught to perceive these traits describe them as I do, makes this phenomenon worth sharing and I present the heuristic that the human body has a universal codification of health, organ by organ, available for anyone to read if they know how. Any similarities between the Kortum Technique and conventional, alternative, or energy medicine methods are coincidental. However, any similarities found may suggest synergy in the collective consciousness of health care and medicine.

Although this manuscript originated from clinical trials, I will deviate from language styles and tropes customary to technical or academic writing. I hold no degrees in medicine and have no formal training in medicine—conventional, alternative, energy, or otherwise. I am purely the cryptographer of a language of health expressed by the human body. I also realize that a completely mental approach will not unlock the doors to many of our medical mysteries, and while medical cures are often found in the laboratory, healing is found in our day-to-day living.

These pages illustrate the discovery of the human body's natural language of health, but this is only one example of our human potential. There are infinite paradigms of perception waiting to be shaped by the human spirit, and in the end, these pages are intended to perspicuously blaze a trail to the gates of perception that you closed long ago and vividly revive the natural sensory abilities that you already possess.

What is the nature of your subliminal odyssey—art, science, music, education, leadership, peace, personal ventures? I cannot say, but this book demonstrates the undimmed power of your perception. Many people consider the uncommon use of the senses as extraordinary or somehow implies enlightenment. However, there are many uses of the senses that are natural to us all yet remain unpracticed. Human sensory perception is simply a prism we gaze through until we refract the reality we *want* to see. Many people seek a life course of least resistance, and once they arrive, they look no further into their prism. My experience has been if you live with passion and a nurturing vision greater than your own and keep turning your prism, you will illuminate your path of purpose. And if you encounter resistance along the way, then it is likely that you are on a healthy course—full steam ahead!

John Christopher Kortum

CHAPTER ONE

The Wind and the Door

MY THOUGHTS WERE far away in the streets and alleys of London as I folded my socks and placed them in my suitcase on a warm afternoon in early November 2001. I had not been to England in quite some time, and I looked forward to my trip with fond anticipation. The telephone rang, and the caller's voice brought my awareness back to my home in Virginia.

"Hello, Mr. Kortum, this is the airline calling. We regret to inform you that your flight to London has been cancelled."—my excitement faded as I sat down on the bed—"We are considering all your options, and we will contact you when we have a new travel itinerary for you."

I informed the voice on the other end that my itinerary would not allow for any changes. Because of my time constraints, I did not have the luxury of being flexible. In the end, my trip to the UK would not be postponed—it would be cancelled.

I looked at my half-packed suitcase and wondered why fate had dealt me the wild card. I had learned to trust interruptive events such as this and knew that travelling was probably not in my best interest, but disappointment prevailed. What could be more important than my adventures in London? I stared at my suitcase disagreeably for a few minutes when I noticed a small piece of paper on my nightstand. It had been tucked in the middle of a large pile of papers that sat for several months next to my bed, but I noticed it only then with its bright red color. Written on the back was the name and telephone number of Dr. Leonard Wisneski, an endocrinologist in Bethesda, Maryland, a physician known for expanding the vision of conventional medicine while increasing the efficiency of the health care delivery system.

"What's the use?" I said aloud, looking at my folded socks and alarm clock packed tightly together in my suitcase as if I was having a conversation with my personal effects. I had already spoken to numerous doctors during the past three years, and it seemed all a waste of time by now. I had come to accept that no one would ever know what I had found thirty years ago, something I felt was of great value—a naturally projected physiological code of health that comes forth from every man, woman, and child.

§ § §

At first glance, there are many obvious physical traits to notice about any human being, and the body's code of health was one more set of perceptible traits to me—obvious but without meaning. Eventually, the events of my childhood revealed that this perceptual code contained comprehensive health information. The reason I call it a perceptual code is because even though it is detected with my eyes, it is not solely a visual perception. I use my sense of sight with certain *sensory adjustments* that allow me to perceive the code. In short, I allow a wider range of information to come to me through my eyes by blending my sense of touch and sense of hearing with my eyesight. Not only do I see with my eyes, but I can also feel with my eyes and hear with my eyes. I know this description of the senses may sound nonsensical, but it is likely there are times when you blend your senses in similar ways. You simply do not recognize that you are.

The code is composed of a set of visual cues that correlate to the body's major organs and systems, for example, respiratory, digestive, reproductive, and so on, and signify when a body organ or system is imbalanced or unhealthy. I call these visual cues *indicators*, and I had spent the last three decades deciphering their encoded content.

For a long time, I had wanted to test the validity of the indicators via clinical research trials. My intention has always been to establish a simple and reliable assessment technique that performed effectively in the health care delivery system. Once established, health care providers could also learn to translate the body's code of health and identify warning signs whenever they met with their patients. Early notification could avert illnesses, and people could maintain their health without interruption. But first, I needed to substantiate the indicators and the technique with confirming medical feedback in a clinical environment. However, this kind of technique need not be limited solely to medical practitioners. I feel that anyone can learn to use their innate sensory awareness to identify these indicators and track their own health and well-being.

What if you could open your sensory channels and receive reliable feedback from your body about your own health or progress of healing? Furthermore, if you could use your senses in such a way that you could detect a physical imbalance *before* it becomes a threat or even manifests in your body tissues, the future of your health would chart a remarkable new course.

One would think that information as progressive as this would be whole-heartedly embraced by the medical community, especially since television and other media channels have recently become platforms for new insights relating to medical treatments and healing. Health care has begun to look over the steep wall of conventional medicine to find effective substitutes to an allopathic approach. According to some media reports, alternative medicine had matured, and that meant more than herbal lotions and home remedies. For the first time, many alternative therapies were regarded as legitimate or at least logically plausible when addressing matters of health. The combined interests of health care providers and health care consumers had finally caught the attention of the public, and the media was there to promote.

I followed along with interest, confident that the perceptual code of health I had observed since childhood had been noticed by medical specialists who see patients every day with similar health complaints. They must have noticed the consistencies between the indicators and the same health imbalances they diagnosed on a daily basis. Surely others had seen these indicators of health, or had they?

Even though I listened to recorded lectures, attended conferences, and watched television programs about transformative health practices, the indicators were nowhere to be found. I had kept this information to myself since childhood, but since the media had presented conventional doctors embracing unorthodox methods, it seemed the time was ripe to act. With only a pocket full of perceptions, I sent up a flare in the night of medical science to share my perceptual code of health with any physician who would listen.

There are obstacles to be faced in every journey, and mine already had its share. I had contacted physicians in Pennsylvania, Rhode Island, Virginia, and Missouri. I had contacted physicians in private practice and university medical schools, even an Ivy League medical school. Setting up a clinical study would be easy, and the process of evaluation would be simple and inexpensive, I explained. All I needed was to look at a patient in their examination room. It would only take a few minutes, and I could render information about the body organs or systems that I perceived were in distress. The results could be quickly tested for accuracy by comparing what I said to the medical diagnoses the physicians already held about their patients. But the conversations never lasted long enough to describe an indicator to a physician. The resistance from the health care delivery system was broad and swift, and I had heard every possible refutation: "Absolutely not, no way;" "that is not possible;" "not with my practice you won't;" "the medical school won't allow it;" "we can't do that with our patients;" and "under no circumstances can you ever meet or have any contact with the patients." Sometimes obstacles can lead to more passion for the pursuit, but I had finally reached an impasse.

Three years had lapsed, and my search for a physician to join me in research was without success. While a few doctors expressed personal interest in my ideas, the norms of the traditional medical profession prevented them from pursuing their individual curiosities. What I discovered beneath the surface of health care was a profession steeped in tradition and locked into a well-established paradigm, a priesthood. And that paradigm was not open to renegotiation or any substantial change.

The most interesting response came from a physician who suggested a clandestine clinical testing method. The study would have to be conducted under certain "limitations" as defined by the physician. I would sit in the waiting room, *disguised as a patient*, observing other patients while they waited for their appointment. I was to take secret notes and then report my observations to the physician after the patients had left. But peering through cut out eyeholes of *Ranger Rick* magazine while appraising the health of patients was not what I had in mind for substantiating clinical efficacy. Although I appreciated this physician's willingness to design a clinical study that circumvented conventional restraints, his approach seemed awkward at best. Besides, medical ethics mandates that patients be aware of their participation in *any* clinical trials. If this was going to be a successful research study, everyone needed to be willingly and knowingly involved in the process, including the patients.

But I did not give up just because I had bumped into some resistance along the way. When I failed to connect with conventional medicine, I went straight to the neighbors and knocked on the doors of unconventional medicine. Since the alternative, new age, or energy medicine communities claimed to hold the keys to healing that went beyond the boundaries of conventional methods, surely I had found a community of practice that would listen.

However, when my model of body indicators did not match their popular trends or commercial wisdom, I found myself staring into the face of new age fundamentalism, if you can fathom such a thing. Although the alternative and energy medicine communities used a different wording, I encountered the same rigid structure of intellectual politics as in conventional medicine. It was abundantly clear that if I was going to bring this medical information forward, I was on my own. But at the same time, I needed a patron in order to progress to the level of medical testing I had envisioned. While most health care providers had retreated, some came to the water's edge, and a few had stuck a toe in, but I needed someone to dive into the pool. The more I thought about it, I knew that not just any health care patron would do. I wanted someone with vision, someone prone to action, *and* someone who also happened to be a physician; I needed a fire starter.

§ § §

Sitting next to a half-packed suitcase, with nowhere to go and holding my passport in one hand and a red piece of paper in the other, I recalled making Dr. Wisneski's acquaintance a year ago. I glanced at my suitcase once more and then back to the piece of paper. Would I have noticed the paper had the airline not called? Perhaps my next adventure was not in London after all, but right here in the palm of my hand. I picked up the phone and dialed.

He remembered our previous meeting and took my call. After we exchanged typical pleasantries, I went straight to the point. "Len, what would you say if I told you that when I look at people I can see their health?"

"Tell me more," he said.

"I have some ideas and perceptual theories that I want to test. The reason I called you is because I am looking for a physician who will test my perception in a clinical environment. If my hunch is correct, this kind of perceptual skill could be made widely available and introduce new ways of identifying the underlying causes of illness. But first of all, I want to determine a measurable level of accuracy."

There was a pause. Like all the others, this conversation seemed to be quickly approaching finality. As the silence continued, I prepared for yet another skeptical response when Len replied, "How do you perceive this health information? You must be doing something more than just looking at people."

"Well, through my eyes, mostly, but then I combine my sense of sight with my other senses of touch and sound. It is primarily visual, so I must look at a person in order to perceive their health. Television and movies work well too. Sometimes photographs can show health depending on how the picture was taken. But my best assessments happen when I am with someone, looking directly at them."

"Oh, so you're an on-site intuitional diagnostician."

"I'm a *what?*"

"You're an on-site intuitional diagnostician," he restated. "Someone like you can use your senses to receive health information in the presence of a person rather than using your abilities from a remote location as others do."

"That is exactly what I do!"

This was the furthest I had ever gone in a conversation with a physician. Unmasking my building sense of excitement, I continued, "Len, if we can get a greater understanding of how I make these perceptions, it may reveal more about understanding human beings and human health. If we are successful, this process could be integrated into the health care delivery system."

Since we had gone this far into the conversation, it was time to get to the point. "Len, I know that you are well connected here in the Washington DC area. Do you know of any physicians who would be interested to join me in a clinical venture? I really want to find out where this will lead."

Again there was long silence in the receiver. I braced myself for the same excuse of why a health study of this nature, although gallant, could not be pursued for conventional reasons, when he said only two words, "I would."

His reply was foreign to me, and before I could respond, he spoke again, "My schedule is very full right now, and we are coming up on the holidays. If you can come to my office on Tuesday, the day after tomorrow at 1:00 p.m., we can meet and talk more about this."

The conversation with the airline echoed in my thoughts, and now it was clear to me why I would not be departing for London that evening.

"Yes, as a matter of fact I am free. I can be there on Tuesday."

"Great, see you then."

I hung up the phone and unpacked my suitcase with a smile.

§ § §

At this point in my development, I did not have a journal or any notes to present to Dr. Wisneski. Everything I had learned was stowed in memory.

But I figured that would be okay because we were just going to discuss a clinical study. Actual testing would come later, or so I thought.

The following Tuesday, I arrived at Wyngate Medical Park in Bethesda, Maryland. Dr. Wisneski had a very interesting professional history. His highlighted specialties included internal medicine, endocrinology, integrative medicine with an interest in psychoneuroimmunology, and medical acupuncture. He was a clinical professor of medicine at George Washington University Medical Center and an adjunct clinical professor of the National College of Naturopathic Medicine. His former positions include founding medical director of the Bethesda Center, president of the Washington Region of American WholeHealth, corporate medical director of Marriott International from 1979 to 1998, and director of medical education at Holy Cross Hospital (a George Washington University affiliate), Silver Spring, Maryland, from 1977 to 1996. Clearly, Len was not just *any* doctor, and of all the physicians I could have found, I knew I was in good hands. The opportunity to work with such an extensively credentialed physician exceeded my expectations.

I entered the office and sat down in the waiting room. Dr. Wisneski approached, and we shook hands. As we proceeded down the corridor, a gentleman passed by us. Len turned to me and asked, "What do you see when you look at him?"

It never occurred to me that I was going to be tested *today*. I thought we would only *discuss* the structure of the clinical study. I hesitated and then replied, "Does he know anything about this?"

"Don't be concerned. I already have his consent to discuss his health with you. He knows why you are here today."

I told Len that I saw an imbalance in the man's digestive system.

"Yes, that's true. He does have a digestive disorder. Hmmm, interesting."

Len opened the door, and we walked into an examination room. Sitting on a chair near the examination table was a middle-aged woman, her eyes full of tears.

"What do you see when you look at her?"

When I looked at the woman, my heart began to pound. Her health was much more threatened than the man in the hall. The tears in her eyes told me she was concerned about her health, and I hesitated to fully disclose what I saw. Obviously, she knew why I was there too and probably would give a lot of weight to my words. What if I was wrong?

When I looked at her, I knew there was more than one aspect of health out of balance, and I was not sure how much to disclose at this point. She demonstrated a combination of imbalances—an obvious breast indicator and a slight blood indicator. Playing on the side of conservative, I chose to address her blood indicator.

"You may want to check her blood." I said.

I was not sure if I should say anything about her breast indicator just yet. But before I could comment any further, the woman stood up, thanked me, and left. Once the door was closed behind her, I looked at Len for feedback.

"From a traditional Chinese medicine perspective, you are right on."

"I don't know anything about traditional Chinese medicine, or any other medicine for that matter. I go by my observations and describe what I see using my own vocabulary."

"She has a lump in her breast, and she's very upset about it," he said.

I regretted not having said anything about her breast because it was obvious the afternoon's events were aimed at establishing my credibility prior to agreeing to any clinical study. I had never been in a testing environment with someone observing my performance, and I was apprehensive, to say the least. "Yes, that's true. She has a breast indicator."

"Can you tell me which breast has the lump?"

I told him.

"But you can tell her that she is going to be all right," I said. "Her Life Span Moisture Level is pretty good, so she should recover in time."

"Her *what* level?" Len asked.

"Her Life Span Moisture Level."

"What's that?" Len asked.

"The way I see health is multidimensional. One way is through the indicators that correlate to each of the body organs or systems. But there is more information than that. There are other factors I call modifiers, and collectively, I receive a whole health picture as well as prognostic information."

"You can see the direction the illness is taking?"

"Yes, the modifiers that accompany the organ indicators tell me about the nature and progression of the health imbalances. *Life Span Moisture Level* is the name I have given to this particular modifier. It relates to a measure of the body's ability to respond to any health threat over the course of a human life. The higher the level of Life Span Moisture, the greater strength the body has to maintain health or prevent disease."

"This modifier tells you how much of a threat an illness is to the whole body system?"

"Yes, but it does not mean that a person is free and clear from a disease just because they have a high moisture level. While a person may have cancer, a high level of moisture usually indicates they will recover. Medical procedures and lifestyle changes may be necessary in the short run or the long run or both, but the level of Life Span Moisture often correlates to the body's endurance."

"What about hers?"

"She may need some treatments or procedures, and she may struggle with her condition in the short term. Based on what I see today, she should be okay. But if her Life Span Moisture Level should change for some reason, it would be important for her to know because it might mean making some changes to her health recovery plan."

"Hmmm, interesting."

The door opened again and in walked a woman in a white lab coat.

"John, I would like you to meet Beth Renné. She works with me here at the office. She is an integrative nurse practitioner and Gestalt therapist."

Beth received her bachelor of science with honors at the State University of New York at Buffalo in 1979 and, in 1984, a master of science in nursing from Catholic University of America. Her practice includes primary care, women's health, and Gestalt therapy, with special interests in psychoneuroimmunology, and natural medicine.

Len wanted a demonstration for Beth, and so another patient was brought into the examination room and sat down before me. I looked at her and described what I saw. "There are a few things going on with her," I said. "For starters, she has a thyroid indicator most obviously. She has a digestive indicator that relates to the upper intestinal tract, not so much the lower or large intestine. However, it is not a serious threat to her system. She also has a reproductive indicator, and there are two kinds of reproductive indicators that I see in women. There is an indicator for when there is an illness and another indicator for what I call dormancy or infertility. In this case, she has the reproductive dormancy indicator." Turning to the patient, I asked, "Have you had any difficulty conceiving children?"

"Yes, becoming pregnant was difficult, and I also began menopause early at the age of thirty-five. I have some digestive complaints that have been diagnosed as irritable bowel syndrome (IBS), but according to my most recent blood test, there is nothing wrong with my thyroid. It's working normally."

The woman left the room. The three of us looked at each other in silence.

"How were you able to know all that?" asked Beth.

I remained silent. I was not sure exactly what to say. The silence continued as I searched for the words because what I said next could make or break their decision about conducting a clinical study. I anticipated that Len and Beth expected an explanation so mysteriously complex that it would reduce the conventions of intellect to confetti. But deep inside, I knew the answer was plain and simple. I decided it was best to explain in very ordinary terminology and said, "Didn't you see the holes in her face? Didn't you feel the dark thickness when you looked at her? Didn't you hear the silence around her?"

Len and Beth exchanged glances and then looked back at me.

"Please continue." said Len.

"Health imbalances leave traces, very distinctive traces. I am using my everyday senses to perceive these indicators. You just need to know what to look for. That's the easy part. But the tricky part is correctly interpreting what you see. I can't fully explain all that I see yet or promise perfection. Many conventional medical tests are not 100 percent accurate either. However, most people continue to place their loyalty in our health care delivery system. Even with the evidence of regular mistakes in diagnosis and procedures. There will always be room for statistical error, but after many years of seeing people's health, I am convinced that these indicators are true. True enough that I came to your office and want you to consider a clinical study with me. If we can provide a scientific basis for how this works, by putting this perceptual process through protocols, we could begin to reveal the body's hidden potential of health *and* human perception. That alone will invite the attention of medical science. But I can't *medicalize* all this for you right now. I don't know how to build a clock, but I do know how to tell the time, and this woman's indicator tells me she has a thyroid problem."

"How can you be so sure?" asked Beth.

"People wear their health like a suit, and it cannot be concealed. The thyroid indicator was one of the earliest indicators I learned to translate because it is so prevalent with women in our culture. It is like a female prostate organ, if that makes any sense to you. I see thyroid imbalances all the time walking down the street. It is such a straight-forward call."

Len and Beth looked at each other once more with questioning glances. It was as though they both knew something that they were not telling me. I continued, "With regard to infertility, I am sure you know of couples who want to have a family. After many years, they find that they cannot conceive a child. This can cause a lot of tension for a couple, especially as they get older because the clock is ticking. If they are unsuccessful, eventually, they may decide to adopt a child, and after they adopt, that is when the woman becomes pregnant. When their focus is withdrawn from the frustration about not conceiving, it is then that conception can actually take place. The reason could simply be that they are relaxed about the whole process because they are no longer invested in a particular result. I know women who say they are infertile because their medical tests suggest infertility if no other cause can be found. But I can look at women and see they are quite fertile. This kind of information might be of interest to some couples who want children. It could bring them relief if they knew there was nothing wrong with their bodies. Then they could focus on the underlying cause of the lack of conception, which is not necessarily biological."

"So you're suggesting that there are other factors that cause infertility?" asked Beth.

"What I have learned over time about these indicators is that the body can demonstrate symptoms with and without an illness. Sometimes there is a delay before an illness shows up in the body, but whether or not there is an indicator, there is always a message behind the body's metabolic behavior to be revealed."

Beth was looking more interested as she spoke, "I have two comments. The first is that this kind of assessment has the potential to be of great benefit to our conventional medical model in many ways. Secondly, implied within your process is the ability to make a distinction between health imbalances that are purely biologically based and those that may be caused by an emotional or even . . . a *spiritual* nature. And if that is true, then it has tremendous implications in the way we develop and implement our patient treatment plans. This information would also be valuable to our patients, for obvious reasons."

"Well, that's why I'm here today. Other than a semester of Zoology 101 in college, my knowledge of physiology and anatomy is limited to common knowledge. I know the basic functions of the body organs and systems, but my explanations about people's health are guided by what the body tells me."

"What do you mean by that?" Len asked.

"Health care uses the language of science to talk about medicine and well-being, but the human body does not. The body has its own language. For example, I didn't identify this woman's thyroid problem by looking for a tired or rundown expression in her face. I didn't look for poor posture or any other physical prompts. I am not distracted by the presence or absence of traditional medical symptoms. I look for a specific indicator somewhere else on the body that correlates to the thyroid. It is the exact same indicator I see whenever I look at anyone who has a thyroid condition. The body's language is consistent. I listen to what the body has to say. In this case, her body also tells me that the location of *her* irritable bowel syndrome is based in the upper intestinal tract, not the lower, even though symptoms may be demonstrated from the lower regions. I know this information may be contrary to conventional methods, but sometimes, symptoms can be misleading and distract physicians from the true source or cause of illness. For example, if someone suffers from chronic headaches, it does not necessarily mean there is pathology in their brain. There are many causes for headaches."

"What else can you tell us about these . . . indicators?" asked Len.

"Many people think I look into the body like an X-ray or MRI, and I can tell you it doesn't work that way. In fact, I don't aim my vision at the area of the body where the organ is located. The information comes from somewhere else. People familiar with alternative medicine speak in terms of chakras and ask me if I see a vertical column of 'spinning wheels' within the body, but those are not the terms I would use to describe my perceptions either. People also ask me if I see an aura of colors above or around the body, but that is not the way that I have come to understand the body's language at all. Colors have nothing to do with indicators. The way most people see an aura is by putting their eyes in an unfocused state or focusing their vision a few feet beyond a person. Compressing the lens of your eyes by squinting and inducing a visual chiffon effect is not what I mean by enhancing your senses. Indicators are not determined by counting freckles on the skin or observing specks on the tongue or iris either. The way I describe this process is that the indicators are generated from within the body and are projected through the skin surface, mostly through the face. But you must also *feel* the indicators when you look at them, which is why you must blend your senses to detect their presence. Some people insist that I am talking about an aura, but that explanation doesn't add up. There is something else going on here, but I do agree that there is a relationship between the body, the atmospheric field immediately surrounding the body, and the indicators."

"Are you talking about synesthesia?" Beth asked.

"Not necessarily because synesthesia only describes the act of perceiving from a multisensory state, but it does not explain how it is done. We all know the eye bone isn't connected to the hand bone, so how is it that I can feel with my eyes? While the debates continue about the possible theories of synesthesia, one accepted standard is that people who experience states of synesthesia do so involuntarily. The difference is that I can do this whenever I want to, so my impression is that there is another field of awareness at work here, but there are two sides of the coin. One side is the field of awareness allows my five senses to entangle and share information with each other. If I compare our everyday perception of reality to watching a movie, we perceive a movie as streaming motion, uninterrupted imagery, the same way we perceive the world with our eyes. But a movie is actually a series of individual still photographs that move past a shutter that opens and closes between the still photographs. The shutter movement happens so fast that we do not see each still photograph. We see only the images in motion. Our perception of reality could be very similar. During the moments when our perceptual shutter is closed, and before it opens and the next image appears, the perceptual capacities of all the senses are temporarily unified in field of awareness both inside and outside of the body. When our shutter opens again and we return to our everyday motion picture of reality, our senses also return to their ordinary positions but carry with them the shared data from the unified field, from the senses. But like the movie, we are not aware of this activity because our perceptual shutter opens and closes so quickly."

Len repositioned his hand against his chin and said, "Please continue."

"People are like Christmas trees with strands of blinking lights wrapped around each one if us. When the lights blink on, our senses are in their ordinary state. When the lights blink off, the awareness of the senses momentarily entangle. There is a continual rebound of information between the body and the atmosphere during the blinks that creates this field of awareness around the body. The blink happens so quickly that we don't notice the flux. For the most part, we have been conditioned to appreciate a Christmas tree only when the lights are on, not off. If the same holds true for our senses and we only appreciate our five senses when they are on, in their ordinary positions, and not when they are off, meaning unified, then 50 percent of our perceptual awareness is never included or gets ignored. That's a significant deficit of information.

"The other side of the coin is that the field of body awareness that surrounds another person is also what sends me the information about their health. When a person's health decides to move in a direction of decay, the process of generating an indicator begins. This can happen before any illness is detectable under a microscope or by a conventional medical examination. The person may not even have any symptoms yet or know something is wrong, but the field of body awareness has already indicated permission to host the illness *before* it occupies the body. When the body gives permission and accepts illness, a conversion process begins. The body's awareness, which is not the same as our own awareness, radiates this thought and stimulates the nearby atmosphere of the body's periphery. In between the nearby atmosphere and the body periphery is a gap, a synapse, an atmospheric modem of thought. The body deposits information in the nearby atmosphere and through this process it arrives at the other end in the form of an observable indicator. There's more to it than I can explain right now, finding the words to describe this is actually more difficult than the act of perceiving the indicators. But the interactive motion of information is a very important distinction to make between what I see and an aura."

"Did you say an atmospheric modem?" asked Beth.

"Another way of saying this is 'thought has sound and sound has form.' When a health imbalance occurs in the body, even if the person doesn't know it yet, it becomes a 'thought' in the body's own mind of awareness. When it becomes a thought in the body's mind, it then has 'sound.' Once it has sound, it takes 'form' and becomes tactile.

"In other words, a thought takes form when it becomes a voice in the mind of the body. This voice has a vibrational texture—it can be felt. The same way when we play music loudly, we hear it but we also feel the sound of vibration in our bodies. This felt property is then manifested in an individual's presence or personal 'thought atmosphere' that surrounds each person. I am not reading minds, per se, but it has to do with interpreting the information that's projected from our bodies and how it stimulates the nearby molecules in the air around each one of us. There is a reciprocal effect because this stimulation of the nearby atmosphere constantly bathes us in our own thoughts that settle back into the body. Again, that is why you must blend your senses to detect the indicators because you actually perceive the individual elements of thought and form. You must learn to see what can be felt and heard. Both the body and the thought atmosphere project and receive information."

Once again, Len and Beth shot glances back and forth at each other. Perhaps I had let too many cats out of the bag, so I shifted gears.

"Some aspects of the thought atmosphere are 'micro' elements, and they change depending on a person's mood. It's likely that you've already had an experience of these micro elements of the thought atmosphere. For example, we all know when a friend is having an off day or is in a bad mood based on certain cues. But there are other 'macro' aspects that remain constant in the thought atmosphere, such as health, that do not change with daily moods or emotions. The idea of an aura is that it travels with us everywhere we go—we generate it. However, our thoughts influence the ambient atmosphere *wherever* we go, whatever space we are occupying at the moment. It may seem like an aura, but it is not. A person's atmosphere contains information about them, but you must learn to recognize it before you can interpret its content. The thought atmosphere contains our living landscape, an accumulation of inner beliefs, attitudes, emotions, and ideas both conscious and unconscious. The living landscape is translatable once you know how to read the elements. Once you learn to distinguish these qualities, you can begin to understand the amazing encoded language of the human body. However, the indicators and the thought atmosphere are not the same. The two are distinct yet coexist."

"So," Beth wondered aloud, "does this thought atmosphere cause health imbalances?"

"I really can't say for sure, right now, but I don't think so. It seems more of a mirror or projection screen for what is occurring both within the body and the intellectual and emotional content of a person. However, I suspect that any changes that occur within the body would be reflected in the thought atmosphere. That could mean a change in the body's biology or a change in the body's mind of awareness. If we could remove the body's permission for illness, we might find what we don't know."

"But how do you adjust your eyesight . . . in order to perceive this . . . thought atmosphere?" Beth asked.

"It's simply a matter of learning how to blend the senses together. When that happens, each one of the senses has a greater capacity to perceive. Blending your senses is not the same as using your senses in unison. Watching a movie and listening to the dialogue is using your senses in unison. This is not the kind of sensory blending I am talking about. What I am talking about is multidimensional, the merging of sensory stimulations, but it sounds more complicated than it really is."

"Are you the only one who can see these indicators?" asked Len.

"Recently, my friend's mother-in-law was in the hospital. The woman was in her nineties and was not expected to live much longer. One night, the hospital called her to say that no family member should leave town right now. The time is near. The nurse said that the mother-in-law has 'the look.' My take is that people already have an innate awareness about the different kinds of information we project from our bodies, but have only learned to identify them in very general terms. I have learned to see about twenty-five different 'looks,' and each one points to a different area of the body. Again, these perceptions are primarily optically based; we are talking about identifying certain visual cues even though there is a larger sensory component involved. Since I do not perceive the indicators out of nowhere, there is a consistent structure of body communication, and that is why I suspect these indicators can be applied to everyone."

"How did you know this information relates to health?" asked Beth.

"I didn't at first. When I was young, I was presented with a large amount of unsorted information. I knew my perceptions meant something, but I was only using my eyes to interact with them. I didn't know they had anything to do with human health until I blended my sense of sight with my sense of touch or sound. As I became more proficient, I focused on the translation of the code and understanding the specific information about each organ or system. The language of indicators is very basic, yet there is a vast amount of detail to learn if you want to become proficient."

"How accurate have these indicators been?" asked Len.

"I've never had a research laboratory environment available to test my accuracy. I am sure there is some error with my interpretation of what I perceive, but it should be easy to test since the organ indicators are pretty straight forward."

"What do you mean?" asked Beth.

"Let's say that you have displayed for me ten different geometric shapes without duplication. For example, there is only one square, one triangle, one circle, and so on. And each day you ask me to look at the shapes and pick out the triangle. Do you think that one day I would miss and select the circle? Or if you asked me to close my eyes and feel the shapes, do you think I would select one other than the triangle? The organ indicators, like the geometric shapes, are distinct. All people have certain physical traits and characteristics, such as height, weight, eye and hair color, and so on, and anyone can see these examples. But once you learn to look beyond obvious physical traits, you encounter another layer of traits, those that project from the body. The indicators are just as observable to me as any person's physical traits, they are out in the open for all to perceive. That is why I am certain that others see these indicators too. They just don't know that what they see has any real meaning. I want to bring the translation forward so people will finally understand what they have been seeing all along. To some degree, our culture has been conditioned through literature, lore, or Hollywood movies that any unusual sensory abilities can't come from the realm of the ordinary senses. Therefore, our culture concludes that anything coming to us through our ordinary sensory channels can't be extraordinary, but that idea is very misleading.

"I've gone as far as I can go walking up and down Main Street looking at people and their indicators. I need to take this to the next level. If I can have access to your patients that have already been diagnosed, I will tell you what I see and show you how this works. You can compare my assessments to your medical records. Since your records probably contain health histories, it may explain more about what and how I perceive. Medical assessments are primarily based in chemical measurements, numeric values, and data ranges, but there are other aspects of health that cannot be counted, that are equally important. Although we can speculate, deep down the big question remains, why would anyone's body give permission for illness to occur?"

There was silence again, and then Len stood up. "Well, I've heard quite enough," he said.

He shook my hand and thanked me for my visit and said good-bye as he moved toward the door. Since my performance was less than 100 percent accurate, I had missed my only real opportunity to be clinically tested.

As Len opened the door to leave, he stopped and turned to me and said, "Can you distinguish between the severities of disease when you look at someone? Lung cancer and asthma are not the same, and to be able to identify the difference is imperative. Find a way to categorize your perceptions so that you can determine the extent of illness in a clinical environment."

"That sounds to me like we are going to have a research study."

"Most definitely, the study will be conducted here at my office. We need to develop a testing protocol, and there are other details to be worked out, such as coordinating office hours and selecting patients, which will take time to organize. We will contact you once everything is in place."

Len removed a folder from a stack on the shelf and gave it to me (see appendix A). "Here are some standard evaluation forms we use here at the office when meeting with patients. "Organize your indicators to match these forms the best you can. It will simplify the study if we can keep both kinds of health assessments compatible."

"Okay, Len, do we need to meet again before the study begins?"

"I am involved in several other projects right now. As you requested, I can provide you with patients and my office as a place to work, but Beth will be the one to work closely with you on this."

Beth nodded.

"She will be the research project manager. Besides, the two of you will make an excellent team."

"There are others who use intuitive methods to assess the body's environment and achieve similar diagnostic result as yours, but I have never heard anyone describe the process the way you have. Could you draw these indicators on paper so we can get a better picture of what you are talking about?" Beth asked.

"You mean make illustrations of the indicators like a blueprint? Hmmm, yes, I think I could draw them for you with some explanation. However, there are a few indicators that cannot be drawn. They can only be understood by showing you because the degree of visibility for each indicator is not the same. The best way to learn is to be in the actual physical presence of someone who has an indicator. If people want to learn how to see these indicators, they need to know what to look for, but they also need to know *how* to look, and that means learning to 'feel' with the eyes. It is more than visual. But if you think illustrations would help to create awareness about the indicators, then I will draw them as best I can."

"You make it sound so easy. Do you think you can teach others how to do this?" asked Beth.

"I've had some ideas about teaching for a long time. I don't think it would be difficult, but it all depends on whether or not people are genuinely interested to see their world in a new way. Our precious beliefs about the way reality *is* are seldom released without resistance. But that is an important step to this perceptual process and teaching people how to fully access their senses. But before I develop a teaching modality, I need to know how accurate this style of health assessment can be. All that I have said is conjecture unless I have the opportunity to demonstrate this assessment model and back up what I say."

"Do you think you can be ready to start in a few months?" Beth asked.

"Yes, but I have no formal education about anatomy and physiology. Do you think I should take some classes first? You mentioned something earlier about traditional Chinese medicine. Do I need to go to China and learn about other medical methods or traditions before we begin the study?"

Len and Beth both shook their heads. They were opposed to the idea.

"Don't try to figure this out from another perspective," Len told me. "Studying physiology and anatomy or any other way might dilute what you can do. If you change your approach right now, it will likely reduce your accuracy. It is important to remain right where you are, with your senses, and we'll see where this leads you. Trust your own process and listen to your own voice, not the words or ideas of others. Leave the physiology and anatomy to me and Beth."

I thanked them and left.

A wind had blown the door of my past wide open; a wind of change and action!

As I walked toward the parking lot, my thoughts were far away into the future of possibilities. Unknown to the three of us at the time, my assessment of the woman's thyroid was not incorrect. It would be several months before a conventional test could detect any imbalance. But by then, it would be too late. She would be diagnosed with one of the worst hypothyroid conditions Dr. Wisneski had ever seen.

CHAPTER TWO

The Powers of Observation

HOW CAN SOMEONE without any medical training or experience, without noting any physical signs or symptoms, without any knowledge of health histories or laboratory values walk into a medical doctor's office and make accurate health assessments merely by looking at patients? My explanation is simple—our perception of reality is negotiable.

In general, we are accustomed to our perception by using certain accepted procedures and techniques. It is true that we are also inherently bound by specific undeniable parameters of our existence. Each one of us inhabits a sentient sanctum called a body, a complex cubby of biological, emotional, and intellectual activities. Our bodies are equipped with sensory receptors (when I use the term *sensory receptors*, I am referring to our five physical senses: seeing, hearing, touching, tasting, and smelling) that allow us to detect sensory stimuli in our environment. Our five sensory receptors are the hardware of our body system that allows us to perceive.

The world outside of our body, otherwise known as the material world, contains substances that we can perceive using our sensory receptors. These substances, such as, sunlight, food, temperature, gravity, plants, animals, other organism, and so on, all have certain undeniable parameters as well. The mechanics of our sensory receptors and how they operate have been explained to us by physiological studies. Our physiological theory tells us what our sensory receptors can and cannot do. In other words, the ways our sensory receptors perform are based upon certain rules—rules of physiology tied to parameters of the material world. By and large, we agree that each one of us plays by the same set of parameters or rules. We all live with the expectation that reality *is* a certain way. For example, when the light turns green, we step on the accelerator, and when the light turns red, we step on the brake. In order for traffic to move in an orderly and synchronized manner, we must also be experiencing the *same exact perception* at the *same exact time*. Therefore, we live with the implication that only one true

44

defined material reality exists—the one that we all collectively perceive. Because, after all, green *really* is green, and red *really* is red.

To one degree or another, all of us are all locked into paradigms of perception that tell us reality *is* a certain way. We rely on our rules of perception because to some extent, our survival depends on it. If we cannot play the game of "green light, red light" correctly when we operate a motor vehicle, we will find ourselves in harm's way.

However, the detection of stimuli in the material world is the beginning, not the end, of our sensory experience. Next, we enter an elaborate cycle of interpretation whereby sensory input is converted into meaning. As our perceptions move through this interpretation cycle, they are subjected to influential ingredients along the way. For example, our personal moods, likes and dislikes, wants and don't wants, and hierarchy of needs get added to our perceptual mix as do social interests and attitudes. This is not a complete list of influential ingredients, and any one or combination thereof can make substantial amendments to our interpretive process; as such, our perceptual product is an amalgamated censorship of reality.

Seldom do we consider our perception of reality to actually be a product, one of many in our consumer driven culture. Economic, social, and political interests often play a significant role in evaluating and prioritizing the kind of reality that we perceive and perpetuate. For example, the world is not flat—it is round. We all know that now, but there was a time when we were not sure or even resisted the idea. This reality was not established in fact because the people of the time wanted everyone to know the truth about the world, and they were willing to risk life to do so. There were competitive economic, social, and political interests to be realized if the world was truly round. In this example, funding and opportunity played a primary role in establishing the reality that the world is in fact round. These concerted interests persuaded the discovery of a new perceptual paradigm. Look at some of the priorities in our contemporary reality and ask yourself if external interests, instead of truth, play a primary role.

Now that we have established that perceptual information is often influenced and organized by external interest and attitudes, we can observe that perception is a stratified and discriminating process. It is important to note that as result of these intricacies, truthful or important data can get discarded simply because it is inconsistent with mainstream interests and attitudes. We have a continuous relationship between the perceptions we encounter every day and this synthesized version of reality. Therefore, a portion of our perceptual experience has actually been predetermined by preexisting *variables* that sway our perception every day.

The end result is that we live our lives from a place of perceptual selectivity. *How* we interpret our daily events influences what we *choose* to observe about our environment. What we *choose* to observe about our environment influences *how* we interpret our daily events. This reciprocal process provides the frame for what we call awareness. *How* our sensory inputs have been conditioned to perform is the foundation for receiving our experience of reality. A perceived reality ultimately locked by rules of perception that have been *persuaded* by a reality-production process that was put in place long ago. If our experiences of reality are actually simulations of truth, then how do we learn to override the default limits and increase our perceptive abilities?

Here is where we begin to home in on the negotiation points of perception. Some of the rules of reality have actually been presented to us in ways that are easier to relate to but do not necessarily represent the truth. For example, with the advent of the electron microscope, we now know that hard rock has far more *empty space* between the solid particles than actual solid particles. Yet we carry on with the notion that rocks are solid even though the truth is they are not. Have we begun to teach our children to perceive the empty spaces when they hold a rock in their hand, or do we continue to draw attention to the hardness? There is a grain of truth that rocks are hard because there is a quality of hardness that we are able to perceive using our sense of touch. This is precisely why I am suggesting to you that reality is a negotiable spectrum because some of these perceptual agreements we prefer to keep; it is just easier to feel the hardness of rocks rather than feel empty spaces. However, I am here to inform you that rocks *are not* really hard. This is a social construct of perception that we have been conditioned to apply when we describe the sensations associated with the experience of holding rocks in our hands.

This is not to say that all social conditionings of our perception are detrimental. Many of our perceptual agreements have useful value; do not forget green light, red light. One measure of any social conditioning is to ask does this perceptual interpretation hold me back or move me forward? In fact, later on, we will rely upon our perceptual agreements when it comes to examining the descriptions and illustrations of the indicators. What is important to recognize is whether the consistent properties within our collective perceptions expand or contract our awareness.

I have made some rather broad brushstrokes across the canvas of human consciousness and the ways that we perceive. This is not a complete evaluation since this text is not intended to be a discourse in philosophy, psychology, and social studies. Instead, we will set our sights on experience and application. But I have presented enough information early in this text to alert you to the fact that locks have been placed in the flow of your perception. The ways we perceive are not necessarily a function of our reality but often a function of our conditioning. Suffice it to say that with so much noise occurring within our sensory interpretation cycle, a portion of the substances that we encounter in our field of perceptions can get censored or go unnoticed.

In order to renegotiate the boundaries of your perception and detect additional information, we are going to have to break some locks. Learning to renegotiate perception is simple but not necessarily easy. Therefore, a certain level of rigor must be attached. The rules of reality will not simply fall away because you say so or because you "think" in a new way. Removing the limits of perception is also an intricate and stratified process. As you peel back the layers of this perceptual onion, inevitably you will encounter competing interests between the locks you want to keep and the natural perception you possess. Real or not, many of your locks have become precious to you, which is why it may be difficult to let them go. However, if you truly want to reclaim your perceptual powers, then forward with breaking locks we shall proceed.

Since your five sensory receptors are the foyers between the external world of experience and the internal world of interpretation, this is where we will begin picking the locks; at the perceptual ports of entry. Except this time we will not hurry our interpretations through a production process. We will slow down our perceptual pace, reduce the noise, suspend judgment, and allow our senses to roam free once more.

Return with me to a time when your world truly was a busy place of wonder. Many of your early perceptual experiences actually had blended sensory qualities. Every sensation you experienced, from the tiny pebble in your hand to the enormous rainbow in the sky, cradled you in awe. Recall standing in the falling rain with your arms stretched open wide as a myriad of tiny comets rushed toward you. You *felt* the *sound* of water splashing against your face as you gazed up into the clouds. You *heard* the *feeling* of rhythm as the rain tapped the streets, the trees, or the rooftops. You *smelt* the *feeling* of moisture penetrating the soil. All of your perceptions merged to create a solitary lens of perception. Remember the sunrise only moments before daybreak. You *felt* the *sight* of dark hue turning to a sea of coral or silver glass in the sky. You *tasted* the *sound* of morning dew as night's velvet curtain lifted to reveal its moisture mark. You *saw* the *feeling* of a soft breeze blowing around you as if miniature fragile feathers combed your skin. You *felt* the *sound* of tiny creatures shaking their slumber to greet dawn's early light. It was a multisensory orchestration of sights, sounds, feelings, smells, and taste raveled into a single expression of perception.

Perhaps your early memories offer similar examples of exploring the range of your sensory receptors. Blending your senses was once natural and simple. However, for many of us, these rich sensations faded with time. We no longer stand in awe about the rain or in amazement about the sunrise. Instead, we are in a hurry to keep our appointments and satisfy our daily tasks. Our attention to the world around us has been substituted for another kind of awareness, an "adult reality" of getting things done, and we no longer behold the magnificent miracles of life. Without continued stimulation for growth, our perceptual tasks become perfunctory or routine. Our net result no longer captures the full range of sensory stimuli available to us.

These liberal ways of perceiving were also natural to me; I did not need to *try* to perceive in this way. It was the way of the world. Even though I grew up in a culture that valued conformity and compliance, I pursued my senses with boundless unity. I approached every activity, marvelous or mundane, with the same level of attention as though they were happening for the first time, every time. Eventually, when I found myself in periods of boredom, I would intentionally bring my senses together as a form of entertainment. It was during these moments that I noticed that people have indicators, projections of qualities that went beyond ordinary physical traits. Although I had no words to explain what I saw, or even what to call them, I knew these indicators held significance. But I had not a clue what they meant until one evening, around the age of eight, when my parents hosted a party in our home. What would have been another dull evening of grown-ups packed into the house became the palette from which I would paint my perceptions for the next thirty years.

During my boredom at the party, I entered this blended sensory state and watched the adults wander back and forth through our home. As the evening came to a close, a gentleman in his fifties arrived. I had not seen him before, nor did I recognize him as a friend of our family. He walked quickly past me to mingle with the other guests, and my attention was immediately drawn to a certain property that he radiated from his body, a property that was not shared by anyone else at the party. I interpreted this as a warning signal, and it prompted me to pay close attention and find the words to describe what I saw. I eventually described his indicator as a salt-and-pepper ash that encompassed his face. I did not *see* a salt-and-pepper ash cloud around him, but it was the texture of his presence that had this quality. (Perceiving this texture I am describing would be similar to perceiving the empty spaces in rock.) I could *feel* it as I *looked* at him. And by feeling it, I could perceive it with my eyes.

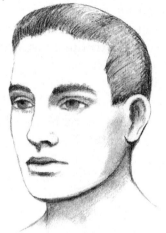
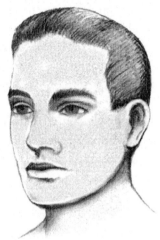

Without Indicator   Respiratory Indicator

The gentleman seemed uncomfortable or upset, and his stay was brief. Once he left, I overheard my parents say he had been recently diagnosed with lung cancer. Unknown to me at the time, I had actually perceived two different pieces of information, a respiratory indicator and a loss of moisture as a result of his cancer, but at the time, it was a single piece of information to me. I would not learn about the distinction between an organ indicator and a loss of moisture until later. The indicator identifies the specific organ, and the loss of life span moisture tells me about the body's endurance and ability to overcome illness. The evening's events were significant because it was the first time I had ever received any feedback about my perceptions. That is when I realized the multisensory mode was not limited to only detecting projected properties—these perceptions conveyed meaning. As I laid my head on the pillow that night, it occurred to me that maybe what I saw related to health. I needed to investigate further, but how?

Evidence could not come quickly enough and was not easy to find at a young age since most adults do not discuss their health problems with children. I had to wait until I encountered another person who had the same salt-and-pepper-ash indicator, which did not occur frequently, and then also find out if they had a respiratory imbalance. It did not matter if the respiratory imbalance was mild or severe; I was looking for any consistency between a distressed respiratory system and an assignable indication. I observed indicators everywhere I went, but without feedback, I could not translate them. My investigation moved into a very long period of watching and waiting.

There was little I could do to accelerate my learning about the indicators. There were few perceptual educational resources available to an eight-year-old child and certainly no resources available to integrate my understanding about perceptions of health. Other than experimenting with my senses and learning how to detect qualities in my environment that others did not seem to notice, my early childhood was that of an ordinary boy. I played sports, was captivated by science fiction, and habitually disobedient. I did not have any lightning-strike events that altered my perception of reality. I simply remained open to all my perceptual functions as my awareness developed and matured; I discounted and rejected nothing.

While I waited to learn more about the body's indicators, prospects were plentiful for recreational perception, and ordinary activities presented tremendous opportunities for growth. While playing on a little league baseball team, my position was in the right field. In case you do not know much about little league baseball, the ball rarely gets hit to right field. I spent many boring hours standing in the outfield waiting for nothing to happen. Since the ball was never going to come my way, I really did not need to pay any attention to the game. Instead, I played with my senses. I was curious to know if this kind of perception could tell me what was *going* to happen. This was not an attempt at fortune-telling, I just want to go a few moments into the future and determine whether or not the player at bat was going to hit the ball—*before* it actually happened. If I could, then I would know when to actually pay attention to the game, given the rare chance a stray ball might come my way.

I observed each batter as they approached the plate for the pitch and *looked* for anything to *feel* about them. I was not looking for athletic confidence, body strength, or proper batting posture. I was looking for any preindications of the instant sensation that the players and crowd *feel* when they *hear* the crack of the bat meeting the ball.

I also observed the batter between pitches as they stretched their arms, walked back and forth from the plate, or took some practice swings. This was my first encounter with the thought atmosphere. In this example, if the player was *going* to hit the ball, I perceived a tactile sensation in the atmosphere surrounding the batter, a knowing in my thoughts, all combined with the visual cue of looking at the batter approach the plate for the pitch. It was as though my eyes had fingers that could feel my field of vision. I made the important connection between the visual cue of looking at the player and the associated feeling when the player was going to hit the ball. If the player was *not* going to hit the ball, the indication was simple—there was nothing to feel. The combined tactile, knowing, visual cue sensation I had established was absent. In this case, my vocabulary began to develop much the same as learning a foreign language, beginning with two basic words, *hit* and *no hit*, in other words *yes* and *no*.

I continued to search for pieces to the puzzle, but oddly enough, the pieces eventually found me. In fact, they came straight into my home and television became my next indicator-learning seminar. *The Tonight Show* with Johnny Carson provided me with nightly perception lessons. As his celebrity guests publicly revealed details about their personal lives, which sometimes included health problems, I finally received the critical component to the translation of the indicators: feedback. I was able to resume the construction of my body organ/system vocabulary as I accurately connected indicator to illness from those who revealed their health histories on national television. However, it was difficult to assign *all* the indicators to the corresponding body organ or system because in some cases, the celebrity guests may not have known they had poor health and, therefore, did not speak about any specific illness. As I matured, this created a dilemma within me. For the first time, sadness and a sense of responsibility were associated with these perceptions. Even though there were times I could not pinpoint the body organ or system in distress, the Life Span Moisture Levels of Johnny's guests were obvious, and I knew instantly who would survive their illness and who would not.

Soon after, the local cinema joined my curriculum and became an adjunct to my television teachings. In those days, *Saturday Night Live* was new to television, and Mel Brooks's productions were popular for creating motion pictures of outrageous comical content. I became a huge fan of both. As I watched the actors on the television and movie screen, I also noticed indicators. I began making comparisons and contrasts amongst celebrities. One of the first important similarities I noticed was that Gilda Radner and Madeline Kahn projected identical indicators. Unknown to me at the time, these two women were teaching me about the female reproductive indicator and the loss of moisture pointing toward cancer. But without any feedback, I had no way of knowing if they had any debilitating health imbalances, or if they knew they did. Although I had some of the indicator translations confirmed, I began to question if my perceptions were really about health at all. Because every Saturday night Ms. Radner was on the television performing Roseanne Roseannadanna, and every few years, Ms. Kahn was in a new film on the big screen, both of them alive and well. Several years would pass before Ms. Radner's reproductive illness became publicly known, and another decade would pass before Ms. Kahn received the same diagnosis of ovarian cancer. I was deeply saddened by the feedback and the news of their health. As much as I wanted to translate the indicators, the means by which the answers came to me were sometimes unsettling.

Music was another favorite pastime, and I was happy to have been bitten by the Beatle bug. I remember watching the movie *Help* and noticing that George Harrison was losing moisture more than any other Beatle. I knew how to recognize indicators in people on the street and on the big screen with some success, but what about inanimate projections? I reached for my album collection and examined the Fab Four on the cover of *A Hard Day's Night*. George Harrison's loss of moisture and his indicator closely resembled the gentleman's at my parent's party, and it was detectable simply from looking at the record sleeve. Mr. Harrison demonstrated the indicator during the mid-1960s, but his health condition would not manifest until nearly three decades later. I rummaged though my other albums and noticed consistency in his indicator and Life Span Moisture Level throughout his musical career. How was it that these body indicators could signal their warnings so early, twenty to thirty years in advance in some cases, before any disease had developed? I wondered if I could calculate a timetable for the indicators and when conventional medicine could detect any imbalance or when people would experience symptoms.

My respect for Ms. Radner, Ms. Kahn, and Mr. Harrison remains infinite. Not only for their contribution to humanity, the arts, and entertainment, but also because they provided me with critical feedback about the indicators at a time when I was close to abandoning these observations forever. If their memory can create imagery in our collective consciousness and facilitate the introduction of this language of health for others to see, then their gifts to humanity are far greater than we ever imagined. In later chapters, when you see the illustrations of the indicators, you may be reminded of people you have seen showing indicators who have appeared in the media.

This was also important because feedback and understanding were finally coming forth, but I needed more information. During the 1980s and 1990s, I traveled the United States and western Europe extensively and met people of many different nationalities. My travels confirmed for me how the organ/system indicators, with some variations, remained relatively consistent within other cultures. Now in my twenties, people shared details about their health in conversation, and that meant feedback. Women, especially, were forthcoming about their health problems. I was finally privileged to the conversations I had missed as a child. I never had to ask either. Women openly shared and compared their health problems and their experiences of seeking ways to correct their health imbalances. Listening to these conversations created another classroom for correlating and confirming organ indicators specific to female health imbalances: breast, reproductive, and thyroid indicators. Since illnesses in these areas of the body are common among women, it was easy to make the necessary distinctions and assign the indicator to the corresponding gland, organ, or system. I was often presented with these same indicators day after day for several years, and it made for very accessible learning.

Shortly after, I went through a phase of rescue. I was a man on a mission, running here and there as the caped crusader of health. I warned everyone about their foreboding biological troubles that I saw. However, throwing health darts at people was about as well received as a ketchup-and-honey sandwich. My reports were met with rebukes or laughter as people assured me they had no health problems. I did not yet know how far in advance the indicators could detect imbalances. Some believed that if I told them they had a health imbalance, that I would "plant the seed in their subconscious and actually cause them to contract the illness." I am not sure about the validity of superstition, but if warning people about their health was subconsciously causing them to contract health imbalances, then why did people contract the illnesses I saw even when I *did not* tell them? If mere words can determine someone's destiny, then I ought to run around and warn people they will have "fulfilling lives of love and gratitude" and force their subconscious to fall victim to such a gratifying and affectionate fate, but I digress. Although I had much to learn about the indicators, I knew that health imbalances do not occur randomly or capriciously or from some momentary negative thought or suggestion. The manifestation of illness is a dedicated process. For the few people who did ask me to tell them about their health, it was for entertainment purpose only. My words were taken with all the gravity of a Chinese fortune cookie. I learned the hard way that this was not the venue to inform people about their health. I returned to the privacy of my observations and quietly developed my vocabulary.

§ § §

Throughout my years of silent surveillance, I wondered what it would take for people to embrace the information their body was telling me about their health. If people truly want to be healthy, then they would want to know *all* the information or would they? The label we have given to health is subject to much interpretation and opinion, but one popular estimation is that if we are not feeling sick, then of course we must be healthy. Well, perhaps not. Although many people reported that they were feeling healthy, when I looked at them, the indicators were telling me another story. I could see that illness was already in the formative stages, but the imbalances had not shown up in a conventional medical exam, not yet anyway. Most people take well-being for granted until they experience some kind of breakdown in their health. But by then, it is often too late to avert the illness and they will have to deal with it.

Yes, we have made great strides in the field of conventional medicine, and the resources available today far surpass what was available to our parents' generation. Yet we often find ourselves with many questions about our health that remain unanswered by medical science. The health care delivery system continues to search for those answers. In the meantime, the most common proactive approach to health and healing we have comes from an "outside in" method. What that means is we regulate the absorption of external substances and activities as a way of internally stimulating the body's health. For example, we avoid caffeine, tobacco, alcohol, saturated fats, red meat, sugar, wheat, and so on and replace them with sprouts, spring water, natural foods, exercise, affirmations, and meditation. Even though some people prefer these diets and activities, the reality is that these lifestyles do not *guarantee* wellness. In spite of following strict fitness rituals, precise nutrition plans, and the path to enlightenment, many people nevertheless become ill.

Subsequently, what people are left with is that health is probability based, and they can only *reduce* their odds of experiencing a health imbalance by tracking their biological inheritance, making proper diet and lifestyle choices, and ultimately *hope* for the best. If this is the spearhead of our knowledge of medical science and wellness, then our command of healthy living is nothing more than a random combination of heredity, option preferences, and crossing our fingers. At the turn of the twenty-first century, one would expect greater levels of medical certainty in the evolution of health care. If there is a categorical explanation for what connects us to health, vitality, and longevity, it remains a mystery.

However, what if we had an "inside out" approach to health? What if the reinvestigation of the multiorgan multiperceptual system living within us revealed the missing clues to our medical mysteries? "What is an inside out approach?" you may ask. We could begin with illuminating the encoded information that dwells behind health maladies, organ by organ, and begin to transform health care as we know it today.

A proactive approach to health would mean to maintain a steady conscious connection with the biological system living within us. If we could develop a deeper and openly communicative relationship with our own biology, we could learn to speak the body's language of health fluently. If we only knew how to develop that deeper connection, we could receive notification and heed the early-warning signs before any health imbalance occurred.

As we search for answers, we could learn to identify when we encounter the body's biological encodings of information that are so precisely calibrated that they activate the body's indicators whenever we stray from our path of integral living. Yet information so elementary in design that it has escaped translation because it cannot be found under the conventional microscope of medicine or scientific rationale. In order to access this encoded information, we must learn to see from a new perspective, not through our mind's eye but through our *body's* eye. Only then can we cast light on the shadows of health.

§ § §

"How can it be that my perception is not fully functional when I am aware of the world around me?" you may ask. Here is a simple demonstration of an everyday visual occurrence when awareness and perception diverge. Have you ever looked for an item in your home, an item that was directly in front of you, in your field of vision, clearly in view, clearly accessible and yet you were not able to see it? For example, you might search the entire house for the keys to your automobile only to finally find them in the first place that you looked. They were in full view the entire time, and yet you did not see them. If you have ever conducted such a household search, you never forget how frustrating it can be. The next time you misplace your automobile keys, you recall the last time that you were looking directly at them and did not see them. So this time, you are patient and diligent as you search. Except, once again, you find that you looked directly at them and once again did not see them. While finding the keys to your automobile may not seem as a very significant event, the point is if something so obvious can be in your field of vision and simultaneously elude your awareness, what about something not so obvious?

The ability to recognize what we have overlooked in our field of awareness holds another key to negotiating perception, and in this case, detecting health imbalances. While increasing your awareness in any capacity is beneficial, I am not talking about increased deductive reasoning as a way of expanding your awareness. I am also not asking you to pay *more* attention to what you *already know*. For example, if someone is limping, even if ever so slightly, signifying they are experiencing pain in their leg, foot, hip, or back, but you did not notice their slight limp before and now you do, this is not the kind of increased perceptual awareness I am talking about. While noticing a slight limp may be useful in any medical assessment, previously overlooked or ignored physical signs and symptoms are *not* body indicators.

I am asking you to pay attention to what you *do not* already know; to place your awareness on your unawareness. If you have not noticed these indicators before, it is because your field of vision lacks a certain perceptual distinction. Like the keys to your automobile, the indicators are there, but they have been eclipsed from view.

§ § §

Let us begin with renegotiating the boundaries of perception by examining how much you can notice about people when you look at them.

As I mentioned earlier, we all know that people have different properties or physical traits that are obvious, such as height, weight, hair color, eye color, and complexion. But look a little closer, and you will find that people have *other* properties. Perhaps you have already seen them and not understood their significance. For example, have you ever noticed that some people appear to you as "wet" or "dry"? Maybe you've noticed that some people appear to you as "dense" or "porous"? These descriptions may seem general, rudimentary, or even ridiculous, and you may wonder how they could possibly tell you anything about health. Actually, these descriptions of the indicator properties relate directly to the female body's genital/urinary functions, respiratory system, digestive systems, and the thyroid gland, respectively. If these examples add more questions than answers for you right now, that is okay. There are more steps and details to be shared.

Because of the way I lent my attention, the events of my youth held profound significance for interpreting the body's language of health. However, the practical value would not be realized until the demonstrations that day in Dr. Wisneski's office. The reason I could easily identify health imbalances with his patients is that the language of indicators is consistent and extends to every human body. Perhaps you have seen some of these indicators already, but they were misconstrued to be physical signs of illness. For example, have you ever observed someone who is gravely ill and thought to yourself, *They don't look so good* or even spoke up and said to them, "Are you feeling okay?" In these noticeable moments, the health imbalance has progressed to a severe condition. The indicators and the body's visible decay have merged and become perceptible through the ordinary use of your senses. The blending of the senses is not required to recognize the body's outward expression of illness. But quite often, at this point it is too late to reverse the course of illness. The importance of identifying the indicators *before* the advanced stages of health decay becomes obvious.

Remarkably, if the body's indicators can be detected early, they often grant enough time to respond to during the introductory stage of illness and, in some cases, *before* the introductory stage. If the woman in Dr. Wisneski's office had been warned that her thyroid was moving toward imbalance, she might have been able to avert or at least minimize the effects of her impending thyroid imbalance. The key to preventative health is to detect indicators before illness can manifest in the body. There have been instances when I have observed the deterioration of health progress aggressively, and death was imminent. But in most cases, the body's language provides us with enough notification to respond if we only heed the warnings.

A popular estimate of our origin is that we are born into this world without an instruction manual. Each one of us must find our way in a wilderness of concepts and experiences convoluted by rules of understanding that may not be accurate in the first place. But what if we actually carry around the open book of our lives for all to read? What if included in those pages is the body's natural way of communicating health information? What if it has been completely overlooked because as I have said before, it is all so incredibly simple? I am convinced that anyone can learn to perceive the body's indicators and interpret their powerful messages.

Irrevocably, we will shape all that we encounter, and so long as we do, then why not shape our perceptions most beneficially. I chose to shape a reality that connects deeply with the body's natural language of health, and so can you.

Prominent Points for Chapter Review

Background

- The realm of observation is more powerful than you think.
- The true powers of observation are impeded by socially accepted rules of the nature of reality.
- Some of the rules that pertain to the nature of reality have been presented in ways that are easier to understand or relate to but do not necessarily represent the truth.
- These rules interfere with the sensory interpretation cycle. Therefore, a portion of valuable sensory information gets censored or ignored.
- Once we are able to recognize and access the overlooked sensory information, it becomes available for our use.

Process

- Notice the unnoticed.
- People have properties.

Practical Application

Wake up early in the morning, approximately thirty minutes before sunrise. Refrain from any of your routine morning rituals: caffeine, tobacco, sugar, food, and so on because these will stimulate your body systems and draw attention from your awareness. If you need something to satisfy the emptiness in your stomach, sip a glass of water or eat a cracker. This is suitable and will not distract you body systems.

Go outside and sit on your porch, steps, or any place of comfort available to you. If none are available, you may simply stand or walk, but do so slowly. This is not intended to be a workout or to raise your body's metabolic activities because that will distract your sensory awareness. Places of natural, not man made, noise levels are best.

A comfortable temperature is desirable for this application. If you need to put on layers of clothing, that is okay, but the outside temperature should not be so uncomfortable that you hurry through the application. Conditions of rain, snow, and winds are okay as long as you are comfortable or have shelter. Other than uncomfortable temperatures, activity in the weather can be beneficial to arousing the senses.

Allow yourself to fully experience what you are experiencing: the sights, the sounds, the fragrances, and the feelings of all that surrounds you. Bring your attention to the earth, the soil, and the grass. Allow your senses to detect the layer of moisture in the air. Combine your attentions, notice what you see and feel at the same time. Notice what you smell and hear at the same time. Notice what happens if you place more emphasis on one sense over another. Allow your senses to overlap and explore their spectral ranges.

CHAPTER THREE

Sense and Sense-Ability

THE CLINICAL TESTING at Wyngate Medical Park began in July 2002. On the first day of testing, Beth explained to me the study criteria and protocol that she and Dr. Wisneski had developed. The patients who volunteered to participate in the study had been mailed a packet containing an introductory letter, consent forms, and a patient-intake form (see appendix B). Each patient was then given an appointment for the in-person assessment procedure. During the office visit, the research protocol was reviewed with the patient, and the consent form was signed and witnessed. I had already created my own customized assessment form based on the medical materials Len gave me the first day in his office (see appendix C). In order to connect my observations with the conventional medical model, we needed a common ground of communication, verbal as well as written. To satisfy this common ground, the indicators had to be assigned to the corresponding conventional medical terminology.

For example, in a standard medical review, some of the body's systems are categorized by criteria that may or may not include a combination of individual organ components: blood/lymph, genital/urinary, respiratory system, gastrointestinal and muscular/skeletal. The way I recorded my observations was converted accordingly. If I perceived a health imbalance in a patient's blood, I reported that the patient was demonstrating a blood/lymph indicator. Each in-person assessment included a conventional medical assessment performed by Beth and an indicator assessment performed by me. Data was collected and recorded for each patient based on the protocol (see appendix D).

I had not met any of the patients prior to the day of testing and met them only at the time I performed my assessment. I did not have access to any information of their medical records. The patients and I could not discuss their current health conditions, medical histories, or lifestyles. I did not have contact or communication with friends or relatives of the patients. Much like my first day in Len's office, I only had a few minutes to make my observations. Afterward, Beth and I conducted debriefing sessions to compare the results from each of the assessment procedures (these sessions were tape recorded and have supported the organization of the conversational text).

As I prepared for the study, I reviewed the many intricacies of the indicators from memory. There were so many details to recall over the last thirty years. Could there possibly be anything I had forgotten? It occurred to me that Beth and I had not discussed every aspect of the indicators. Before I met with the first patient, I took Beth aside and told her there was more information that she needed to know.

"Beth, before we start, you need to know more about what I can do, what I can see. It's not black and white. It's not cut and dried. The indicators usually tell about health imbalances that are impactful, long-term, or severe in nature rather than short-lived or minor health problems."

"Do you have a sense of why that might be?" Beth asked.

"Well, health imbalances must reach a certain threshold for the organ indicators to become activated. If you caught a cold or twisted your ankle on the way to the office this morning, it probably would not register in my field of view because that kind of health imbalance would be inconsequential to the body's consciousness. However, if you suffered from continuous respiratory infections or joint discomfort, it would most likely activate an indicator, and I would see it. Likewise, if someone is on the verge of a cardiac arrest with no symptoms or prior history of cardiovascular disease, the indicator would most likely be present. I am not exactly sure why that is, but I suspect it is because the body's consciousness of the disease has been affecting the organ system for a long time regardless of what conventional medical measurements can find."

"Why would that be true?"

"As you know, the human body is subject to all kind of bumps and bruises along the way. The body's indicators seem to only communicate health imbalances that are of real consequence. For example, reduced visual acuity with age is not considered an illness to the body. Some people may need to wear glasses or contact lenses to see objects at a distance or close up, but the accompaniment of an eye indicator for this kind of condition is not likely. Imbalances that affect the health of a person are the ones that activate the body's indicators and subsequently cause the indicators to become observable. How the body determines which imbalances matter and which ones don't, vary from person to person and remains a mystery to me."

"So we need to keep that in mind as we go through the study," Beth replied. "As a scientist, I have one concern, and that is in order to create a valid research study, it is important to maintain consistency and objectivity. Therefore, if you are going to register a 'hit' in this study, when we compare the two assessments, there must be a parallel result. When there is a conventional diagnosis for a certain body organ or system, you must also report an indicator for the same organ or system. If you report an indicator and there is no conventional diagnosis, that is a miss, and if you do not report an indicator and there is a conventional diagnosis, that is also a miss."

"Okay, that sounds fair to me, Beth."

She stood up and left the examination room to meet the first patient. I sat quietly and stared at the stethoscopes, specimen jars, and cotton swabs. It occurred to me that my long-anticipated term of testing had officially begun. A journey that began when I was eight years old and a man with a respiratory indicator walked through my house had come to fruition.

The click of the doorknob brought my awareness back to the examination room. The first patient, Susan, walked in. We shook hands, said hello and she sat down in front of me. As I fixed my eyes on her, there were several organ indicators staring back at me all at once! This was unusual for me to perceive so much from one person. The health imbalances were not severe but present nonetheless. I presumed that my apprehension about the first day of testing was causing my perceptions to exaggerate. I took a deep breath, closed my eyes, and relaxed for a moment. I expected to regain clear indicator vision when I resumed my observations and find only a single organ indicator present. But when I opened my eyes, the same collage of indicators was staring back at me. There was no mistaking what I saw. My concern switched to panic. After years of preparing for this moment, searching for physicians, and all the time and work Len and Beth had devoted to the clinical study, now my vision was blurred? I sat speechless while my heart pounded. Susan squirmed in her seat and then looked at me and said, "Is that it? Are we finished? I didn't feel a thing." At that moment, I blurted an incomprehensible sound. After that, all I could do was laugh. Then she laughed. Then we both laughed, and so I proceeded.

Patient 11013: "Susan"

* Pseudonyms have been used for all patients

John: It might sound strange, but there's a lot going on with her. I had to focus on each indicator one at a time so that I could see them all. There aren't any serious health threats happening for this woman although there are some mild imbalances that I can tell you about. There is a mild ENT (ear, nose, and throat) indicator although there isn't any loss in her ability to hear. There is a mild gastrointestinal indicator, and it specifically relates to the process of digestion, a mild neurological indicator in the head/brain region, and a mild muscular/skeletal indicator.

Beth: This patient has conventional medical diagnoses that include chronic sinusitis, irritable bowel syndrome, food allergies and lactose intolerance, head trauma from a motor vehicle accident, osteoarthritis, temporal mandibular joint dysfunction (TMJ), and many surgeries including the knee and nose. That's pretty good. You hesitated as if you were questioning your perceptions at first. Although your information is general, your report is pretty much on target. You really need to trust yourself and what you see. Don't worry about perfect accuracy right now. We are in a discovery process. Of course, that means gathering data about the patient's health. But that also means gathering insight to how your technique works. If you're too concerned with getting a hit, you might hold back information we can use later when we evaluate the data for consistency.

John: I had assumed that all the patients in the study would only have one health imbalance to detect, but you and Len are going to challenge me. The patients might have many health imbalances. I thought my signals were crossed at first, but your examination confirms what I see. What's peculiar about the muscular/skeletal indicator is that it speaks as a whole system instead of telling me exactly which muscle or bone is affected. The combination of osteoarthritis and the knee surgeries have been converted by the body into a single indicator.

Beth: Okay, so what you are saying is that there is no distinction through your assessment between specific parts of the body system. The body organs speak to you as a whole, and while you may see a cardiovascular indicator, you won't know if the problem exists in the left or right ventricle or if it is a conduction defect."

John: That's probably true, but right now, we are verifying how accurate these indicators are for identifying which body organ or system is in breakdown. I did not say this information is intended to serve as a directive for surgical procedures.

Beth: If all that you are telling me is true about this system of indicators, then this is about bringing forward a new form of health assessment; a way to derive a comprehensive portrait of wellness. Any process that tells about health without invasive and expensive laboratory procedures or delays waiting for clinical test results would be really useful, but I want to know if this assessment technique can provide me with better scientific information than I already have access to thru conventional medical procedures.

John: Sounds like there may be more than one study to be conducted here. All that I have told you, so far, is what I have learned on my own. I've never had clinical technologies at my side to develop my perceptions. This is only my first day of testing. Let's see what happens next.

After seeing the first patient, I knew that Len and Beth had other interests surrounding our study, but I was not sure exactly what that meant. My intent was to get the best overall score during the clinical testing, but they wanted the minutia; they wanted to know every bit of medical detail that I could retrieve. They were looking at a much bigger picture.

Patient 16002: "Heather"

I had a similar experience with Heather. There were so many health imbalances that I had to discern each of the indicators from the mélange that projected toward me. Furthermore, since I had optimal health my whole life, the experience or even the idea of having so many health imbalances was absolutely foreign. However, this presented more learning opportunities as I began to sort and separate individual indicators from a mixed group.

John: There's a lot going on here. Once again, I feel my perceptions must be skewed. How can someone actually have this many health issues occurring all at once?

Beth: Let's not judge or overinterpret the data before it's reported. Just tell me what you see. It's really pretty common for people to have multiple coexisting medical problems.

John: I saw several indicators for this patient. They are all mild in nature, but there are some other things I am noticing: There is an ENT indicator, and in this case, it *does* relate to the patient's sense of hearing (whereas with the previous patient who had an ENT indicator, there was nothing wrong with her ability to hear.) There is a blood indicator. However, there are two different kinds of blood indicators that I see. One category is when the blood has an illness, such as leukemia. The other category is when the blood is a carrier of an illness. There is no pathology in the blood components, per se, but its contents are somehow compromised. For example, this indicator can relate to anemia, cholesterol or glucose levels, and so on. With this patient, the blood indicator is a carrier, and this patient is specifically demonstrating a mild diabetic indicator.

Beth: So what you are saying is that when the blood is a carrier of an illness, the blood is not the bottom line issue. There is a dysfunction somewhere else in the body organs, but the blood condition is where the symptoms come from. The conventional medical diagnosis of diabetes is made by measuring blood sugar, not through the evaluation of pancreatic function, which is the organ that produces insulin. Likewise, elevated cholesterol levels are determined by blood assay, and not by evaluation of the target organ that may be the cause.

John: Well, that makes sense because I detect diabetes in the blood rather than through an organ. It is mild in this patient right now, but it could progress and become more pronounced in the future. There is also a genital/urinary indicator, but it seems as if her reproductive condition was more active in the past.

Beth: How do you know that?

John: When a health condition has passed, it often leaves what I call the shadow of the indicator, a scar. Much like scar tissue, it is the residual effect of trauma.

Beth: What exactly does that mean?

John: The body's language of indicators has a way of accounting for its health history. What I see when I look at this patient is the residual mark of when her reproductive system *was* compromised in the past.

Beth: All right, is there anything else you noticed about this patient?

John: This patient has a mild breast indicator, but it does not look like the condition will progress.

Beth: How do you know that?

John: The indicators also have a level of intensity to them; this intensity tells me whether or not a condition is going to get worse.

Beth: So there is some kind of range that would describe the severity of each health condition. What else did you notice?"

John: She has a mild muscular/skeletal indicator and a mild gastrointestinal indicator. That's it. That's all I have to say about her.

Beth: Okay then, in terms of conventional medical diagnoses, we know this patient has acute ear pain, sinusitis and bronchitis, elevated blood glucose and anemia, had a hysterectomy for ovarian cysts, has microcalcifications in the left breast, and has muscular back pain, joint pain, and tendonitis in the left shoulder. But there is no history of gastrointestinal problems.

John: It is a mild digestive indicator. The body tells me the indicator is present even in the absence of symptoms or the confirmation of a conventional diagnosis.

Beth: So we are talking about intensities again. Your perceptions can corroborate the medical history that I already have for this patient, which may indicate reliability and validity. Not only that, but the indicators also present information that may hold clues to potential risk factors that can be used in a preventative health setting. I am really interested to see how we will be able to use this information in the health care structure as we know it. I wonder how these indicators fit into what we already know. Do you see how much potential this has?

John: It never occurred to me that your patients would have so many conditions to identify. I expected your patients to have only one or two health imbalances to target in the study. There's a lot of stuff to sort out now that I have access to medical records. Especially with you sitting here and asking me questions, we are probably going to find more holes in my vocabulary that need filling.

With our protocol in place, we had not considered that the study would begin to pull our interest in many directions so quickly. Beth and I juggled several questions without apparent answers while my assessment of patients continued with similar results. My descriptions of the indicators seemed somewhat general to Beth as a clinician. She wanted more details from me, and it was not long before the lack of detail presented both challenges and opportunities. However, an inherent limitation dawned on me. Although the indicator vocabulary I had compiled, up until that time, correlated to the different body organs, I had not been witness to every disease possible. There are thousands of different health problems, and that presented the opportunity for the study to go beyond just testing the indicators for accuracy. In view of the fact of unlimited access to feedback from the patients in the clinical trials, I could work on expanding the indicator vocabulary.

§ § §

By the early '90s, I had correlated many of the body organ/systems with their respective indicators, but not all of them. The blood indicator had been easy for me to identify, but with so many possible imbalances in the blood, I wondered if there could be more to it than a single blood indicator. Much like the frequent occurrence of thyroid imbalances, diabetes is common, and I had a hunch the blood indicator might have a specific way of communicating diabetes—a blood indicator but with a slight or unique variation. The evidence I had been searching for eluded me for several years. Then one day, an idea came to me.

I had been working in the international travel industry for many years, and I prepared and served food in a variety of ways to large groups of people. Often I served groups of two hundred people for breakfast, lunch, or dinner, and it was not unusual for guests to request special dietary cuisine. On one such occasion, after preparing the afternoon meal and prior to serving, I reviewed the guest roster for any special requests and noticed that one gentleman had requested a diabetic meal. I wondered if perhaps health information could be translated in reverse order. Rather than observing an indicator and then waiting to find out if the person had a health imbalance, perhaps it could be translated from the other direction. What if I knew the organ or system was already out of balance, and from there I could identify the indicator? It made perfect sense to me and what would have otherwise been a routine afternoon of work revealed the lost key to identifying diabetes.

Once all the guests had arrived, I reviewed the seating assignments and determined where this particular gentleman was seated. I introduced myself and engaged in a conversation long enough to conduct an indicator assessment. All I needed to do was identify a "property" that was new to me. Since I had identified most of the indicators already, I looked beyond the ones he had that I already knew, and through the process of elimination, there it was—the body's way of communicating diabetes.

So that's it! I thought to myself. *Interesting, it was not what I would have expected.*

But I also knew that an organ/system indicator is seldom established by a single individual's projection. This gentleman had provided me with a template, and now I needed confirmation.

During the next few months, whenever someone requested a diabetic meal, I made sure to meet with them personally. After observing the same "property" demonstrated by five or six people with diabetes consistently, I concluded that I had properly translated diabetes.

However, once I confirm any indicator, I never consider it set in stone. I remain vigilant to make sure the indicators maintain their reliability over time, even today. Otherwise, a misinterpretation might occur. On one occasion, I was reviewing the guest roster, and once again, someone had requested a diabetic meal. By now, I did not need to move in closely and speak directly with any guest who had diabetes. I could identify the imbalance from a distance. Once everyone was seated, I glanced in her direction just to make sure, but to my dismay, she did not project an indication of diabetes. I figured the information on the seating chart must be inaccurate, or perhaps the guests switched seats without my knowing it. When I approached the woman and confirmed her identity, I became concerned. Had I been tracking another health imbalance all along believing that it was the indicator for diabetes? The correlation had been reliable and consistent up to this point, but I had to investigate. I intentionally lengthened our conversation to learn what I could from her. At this point, I was looking for any kind of indicator, but I kept coming up with nothing. Even with the disappointing internal conversation going on within me, I spoke calmly to the woman and informed her that the proper dietary arrangements had been made for her meal.

Finally, I was running out of words, and I needed to move on and give my attention to the other guests. But before I left, I asked her if she needed to eat by a certain time with regard to her insulin schedule when she announced, "Oh, I am not diabetic."

"You're not!?" I shouted.

"No, not at all. I have been to several of these dining events with my friends who *are* diabetic, and the meal they received always looks so much better than what was on the menu. So I decided to request one for myself this time," she said.

I was relieved by her news, but it made me wonder how many other indicators I had misinterpreted along the way because of such ambiguities. For example, when people say that they are lactose intolerant, is this a self-diagnosis or have they clinically confirmed their lactose intolerance? I have met several people who claim to be lactose intolerant, and I have not observed a gastrointestinal indicator. In the past, I deferred to people's health claims as an official diagnosis, but I began to consider that the indicators might be more reliable.

§ § §

One day I showed up at the Bethesda office at my usual time, but before we began, Beth wanted to speak with me privately. "John, do you recall the first day you came to the office and you told Dr. Wisneski and me that the woman had a thyroid indicator, and her tests were all negative?"

I nodded. I knew what was coming.

"Well, her thyroid disease has just appeared in our conventional tests. Her symptoms are profound. As a matter of fact, she has one of the most severe hypothyroid conditions Dr. Wisneski has ever seen."

"How is she?"

"She is on medications and starting to stabilize, but it will probably be a long process of recovery. Len is treating her. That is really all we know right now. We only found out a few days ago."

I reminded Beth that sometimes the indicators will appear in people who are healthy at the time of observation, and the physical illness will manifest later. "It has been approximately eight months since that first day in our office and you last observed this woman. That was a while ago."

"People can demonstrate indicators for quite some time before the illness can be perceived by standard medical procedures, so I am not surprised by the news. I clearly saw an indication that something was wrong on that day. If you remember, I wouldn't back down from my assessment even though her conventional tests didn't show any indications. So far in the study, you have heard me use the word *mild* when referring to the severity of a patient's indicator. That is because their health problems have not been life-threatening illnesses, or the problems were much more active in the past, or corrective procedures have caused them to subside. The reason I stayed with my assessment of her thyroid was because she was already demonstrating an intense level of indicator activity."

"How often do you observe people with an indicator but without conventional symptoms?"

"I am really not sure because without feedback, I can only wonder. I see people with indicators all the time at the grocery store or the movie theater. But since I am not acquainted with any of them, I have no way of confirming their health status. Believe me. It does not go over well to approach strangers about their health, or even people I know for that fact. I stopped doing that a long time ago. I had assumed that I was seeing illness in real time and that people already knew about the health issues they had. Or if they didn't know, they would find out soon enough. But now I have learned that sometimes, the indicators can show in the very early stages of illness; which was the case with this woman's thyroid."

"So you really have no idea just how far in advance an indicator can show up?"

"Some indicators are mild, some are severe, and there is a range in between. Your question reminds me of a friend of mine named Reese. She demonstrated a loss of moisture that looked like a rather aggressive cancer, but that was more than ten years ago. I never said anything to her about it because I didn't want to alarm her unnecessarily, especially when I was uncertain about my level of accuracy. We see each other from time to time, and she never said anything to me about her health. We know each other well enough that she would tell me if she had any kind of illness. I often wonder about her health though. It has been almost five years since I last saw her. I want to become as accurate as I can at seeing the indicators, but this is one time I really want to be wrong."

"How does cancer appear to you?"

"It's interesting actually. We've talked about the modifiers and the Life Span Moisture Level the first day I came to your office. The level of moisture relates directly to how successfully a person's body can respond to any threats to their health. I am sure you have heard of two people who have been diagnosed with identical cancers. They both receive the same treatment, yet one goes into remission and the other succumbs to the disease. Why is that so? There are some medical theories that address this question, yet I have noticed that the moisture level can tell you a great deal about what the outcome will be."

"So, what you're saying is that the body has a way of communicating its consciousness, what it knows, about the cancer through the Life Span Moisture Level modifier."

"Yes, it tells more about their recovery forecast."

"It sounds like we are moving into areas that are deeper than conventional medicine can explain."

"Something else I have noticed is sometimes there is a loss of moisture with an accompanying organ indicator, and there are times when there is a loss of moisture without an organ indicator. In those cases, I am assuming that an aggressive illness is moving around somewhere in the body system. It just hasn't selected a place to land yet."

"Really? That would be tremendously useful in identifying primary and secondary cancer sites and subsequent treatment protocols. What does this moisture level modifier look like?"

"Well, when moisture loss is in the introductory stages, you need to combine your senses to detect it, the same as with indicators. When moisture loss is in the advanced stages, then the ordinary use of your eyesight is usually enough to see it. Sometimes people can live for awhile with a significant loss of moisture. But when it comes to health recovery, a high level of moisture can make all the difference."

"It's interesting that you say that because years ago during my medical training, I worked in a cancer ward. I could tell just by looking at people when they were in the end stages of their disease. At the time, I didn't know what to make of the information, but it was pretty clear."

"How could you tell, Beth?"

"There was something I noticed in their complexion, but there is more to it than that. It's as though there was an 'arid vacancy.' The body tissues were lacking in something . . . I can't quite put my finger on."

"Well, it seems we both have a way of describing the body's Life Span Moisture Level and its measure of overcoming or surrendering to illness. It's funny to hear you talk about it because now you know how challenging it can be to find the words to properly describe what you can perceive. It's not so easy because sometimes the words just aren't there, but you must find them. Maybe you can tell me more about your own observations, and we will compare them to what I already know about the indicators."

As the clinical trials progressed, I relaxed about my performance. I dared to make my observations much more specific at the risk of lowering my test scores. Since the body speaks its own language, and not necessarily the language of science, I had to explore these "biophonetics" to increase the precision of my perceptions. My descriptions did not end with stating, "I could see an indicator for a particular organ or system." Now it became a matter of how much detail I could retrieve. While exploring these intricacies answered some of our questions and extended the reach of this visually based assessment tool, the lack of a clear vocabulary slowed our research. Although we were able to gather more medical data from the indicators, we did not have the words to describe what we found.

Patient 01011: "Bill"

John: This patient has a mild genital/urinary indicator. There is also a blood indicator, and right now, it is more than a mild one. In this case, the blood has no illness—the indicator points to blood pressure.

Beth: Okay, the medical history reveals that this patient had a vasectomy and then a reversal. That's interesting because the patient does not have an overt illness in the genital/urinary region, but instead, a surgical procedure was performed. Are you able to perceive past surgeries?

John: I am not sure about surgeries specifically; basically, indicators tell me whether or not an organ or system is in its normal condition. Here, the genital/urinary region has somehow been altered from its natural state, just as any health imbalance alters the body from its natural state. The body is indicating to me that there has been some kind of change to the genital/urinary region. I suppose I have always interpreted an indicator to mean there's a health imbalance or illness, but perhaps what I can see is an indication if an organ or system's natural condition has been somehow altered, most often due to a health imbalance, but it may not be the only cause. Don't forget, an indicator can show up before an illness does, so does the body know about the alteration before it occurs?

Beth: I have always been sure on some level that the body is aware, or has a consciousness, when it has experienced surgery or injury; the body demonstrates this awareness through pain and other signs and needs time to recuperate. But the indicator language takes that intuitive sense to a deeper plane. Not only does the body have a consciousness to respond when it is offended, but it actually has an inherent ability to *voice that fact* as well. This could open up infinite new doorways toward understanding the human body as an interactive entity."

Each patient assessment brought forth new information, but it was not always confirming. In all fairness, I need to present the misses as well as hits. Not every test session had the same level of accuracy. There were the occasional assessments that left us with many unanswered questions. Again, it was another opportunity to increase our learning curve even if that meant decreasing my accuracy score.

Patient 12018: "Loretta"

John: This woman has an entire collection of mild indicators. They are gastrointestinal, genital/urinary, blood that relates to sugar levels, breast, thyroid, and a muscular/skeletal indicator. The breast and muscular/skeletal indicator seem most active to me.

Beth: She has migraine headaches, a history of rhinoplasty [nose recon-struction], and fibromyalgia. Currently, fibromyalgia is considered a muscular/skeletal imbalance, so that is a hit, but the others you mentioned have no conventional medical diagnosis. There is no cor-relation. You are sure about all these other indicators?

John: Yes, but again, they are all very mild.

Beth: For the purposes of the clinical study, this session is not as accurate. You said there were six imbalances, but conventional medicine has only identified one. I suppose, however, that these mild indicators could be potential problems, not yet manifested? Still, we can't consider them until or if they actually appear.

John: Well, yes, I suppose the future might reveal more.

Beth: She also has a history of tobacco abuse, but she has not been diagnosed with any respiratory problems. You didn't report a respiratory indicator.

John: You just said she does not have a diagnosed respiratory condition, so that may be why she does not have an indicator. All I can say is that some people who use tobacco may develop health complications or even cancer. Or if they do develop cancer in the throat or lungs, tobacco is labeled the guilty culprit. But I know people who use tobacco regularly, and they don't have lung cancer or emphysema or any other respiratory complications.

Beth: At least not at the moment, they don't. We can't be sure until their life completely plays out.

John: Do you assume that anyone who smokes will have a respiratory indicator?

Beth: We all know those stray people who are not affected by it, or so it seems. The vast majority of people do compromise their organ functions, but there are some who also have heart attacks from tobacco use. Could your indicator system make a distinction between these two?

John: I think so because an indicator is an indicator to me. I don't include information about person's lifestyle when making assessments. What I am saying is there isn't a one-to-one correlation between tobacco use and cancer or any other habits and cancer for that fact. What about the life of George Burns? He enjoyed both tobacco and extraordinary longevity. And don't forget, there are many people who develop lung cancer that have never used tobacco products. I am not saying that tobacco use is ideal, but the absence of an indicator here with this woman tells me it is not going to be of consequence. Maybe an indicator will show up later, but for the time being, it's not an issue. And even if there was an indicator, I would look to the Life Span Moisture Level modifier for more information. When I see people with respiratory indicators *and* low levels of moisture, that is when I would be concerned. Otherwise, it's usually not a big deal.

Beth: Hmmm, so we have established that not everyone who smokes has a respiratory indicator, not even a mild one. Is that correct?

John: Yes.

Beth: But there are some people who may not have overt chronic lung disease but whose lungs are still irritated by the smoke; maybe they will develop a transient cough or wheeze a little, but their overall lung function is not compromised. Would these people have a respiratory indicator?

John: That is probably why most people, including health care providers, have overlooked these indicators because they make assumptions about the cause of illness and patient behaviors or lifestyles. What do you call a physician who specializes in respiratory illness?

Beth: A pulmonologist.

John: Okay, so let's say you are a pulmonologist. Perhaps the reason you don't see the respiratory indicator is because only *some* of your patients who use tobacco will have an indicator. Therefore, you would not notice any consistencies when you met with *all* your patients who use tobacco. You would assume tobacco use affects everyone's respiratory system the same way, and that may not be true. Likewise, not all your patients are going to die from their respiratory problems. Some people would have higher levels of moisture than others. Furthermore, if your patients have other imbalances occurring at the same time, as some of the people in the study have, then the multiple indicators would cloud your view from the respiratory indicator. To your eyes, the indicators and the Life Span Moisture Level would be even more difficult to distinguish. Aha! This could explain why people don't see the indicators—their intellectual assumptions combined with multiple indicators and varying degrees of those indicators cause each patient to look uniquely different to them. They wouldn't identify any similarity!

I have mentioned several times that the body indicators are simple in their appearance. They are not sophisticated or complex by any means. However, the logic behind the indicators is not the same as our conventional medical approaches. For example, when taking an X-ray, the technician focuses attention on the area of the body where information is desired. While the body has its own rationale, the body's perspective does not always equal the kind of rational format we would expect. The location of the indicators on the body and the area of the body where the correlating organs are found are not the same. For example, when evaluating a thyroid, I do not look at the location on the throat where the gland is located to receive information. The thyroid indicator is projected from the cheeks of the face. In fact, most indicators project from the region of the face. Here is another intellectual fork in the road and yet another perceptual point of negotiation. If we evaluate the body's indicator logic through the lens of our conditioned academic judgment, we will distance ourselves from the body's wisdom and the unsolved mysteries of health and healing. However, by unfolding the body's blueprint of indicators with intellectual grace, we may finally read from the text of our native biological manuscript.

Once you accept the body's form of logic, it is easy to follow. In most cases, the indicators are individually coupled to the organs they are assigned. For example, the thyroid indicator only tells you about the thyroid. However, there are some indicators that point in more than one direction. For example, the blood can relay information about a blood illness and also about the quality content and viscosity of the blood. Another one of these multimeaning indicators is the ear indicator. The ear indicators can reveal information about the condition of hearing, and the indicator can also reveal information about the sinuses or other conditions such as TMJ.

§ § §

Some of the patients sat quietly while I made my observations and then left the examination room after the assessment was over. Other patients expressed an interest to hear what I had to say to Beth about their health after the assessment was over. When the three of us sat together, Beth and I had the opportunity to hear feedback from the patient's perspective but only after my perceptions were recorded for the study. If the patient was present during these conversations, I spoke in general terms of biological "activity." For example, if I observed an illness in the digestive system, "activity in the digestive system relating to lower tract" was the extent of my description in front of the patient. After the patient had left the examination room, I discussed more details with Beth about the activity I noticed during the assessment. My observation also included any prognostic information I may have observed. I wanted to demonstrate for Beth how my technique could provide a clinician with more information than what is ordinarily available through conventional testing or evaluations.

During one of our clinical testing sessions, I observed a patient demonstrating an ear indicator and the activity related to her ability to hear. Beth reported that all conventional tests showed her ears were working properly. While we discussed the results of the indicator and conventional health assessments in the presence of the patient, the patient interrupted our conversation and said to us, "My hearing has been giving me a lot of trouble. I haven't been able to hear very well in one of my ears during the past several months, and it's getting worse."

I looked at Beth, but she shook her head and said, "All of her hearing tests are all normal. Conventional medicine does not confirm any imbalance—that is not a hit."

It occurred to me that the patient's testimony could be more valuable than what the conventional test could show at the moment and should be included in the health evaluation in some way. Beth acknowledged the value of the patient's own testimony. However, she reiterated that since all conventional tests could find no reason to explain the hearing loss, without a conventional diagnosis to confirm a hearing loss, my indicator assessment would not be registered as a hit based on the protocol of the study. Incidences such as this occurred more frequently as the study progressed, but since my indicator assessment consistently detected imbalances based on patient feedback, not conventional evaluations, it caught Beth's attention. After more occurrences, we decided that we could no longer suspend the weight of this observable fact. It needed to be considered, but we were not sure how.

On days when I showed up at the Bethesda office and the patient had canceled at the last minute, Beth and I made use of our free time together. We reviewed assessments that were completed earlier in the study with the growing perspective of the indicators we had gained over the months. During one of these review sessions, Beth made an important discovery.

"John, you have made several references to mild during the study with these indicators. Exactly how mild is mild? Perhaps it is time we developed a measurable or quantifiable scale of intensity to better describe what you can see?"

"Hmmm . . . Well, okay, but how are we going to do that? Won't it be subjective? If I am the one that determines whether an indicator is mild or severe; it's based on my perceptions. I have learned how to determine intensity over the years, but it is still from *my* point of view."

"Well, that's okay. Since you have established the indicator vocabulary, you are probably a good source to determine the range between mild and severe. Tell me how you describe these intensities. Just let your words flow."

"Okay, to the best of my understanding . . . in the conventional medical model when a health imbalance reaches a certain level of intensity, it becomes detectable through medical laboratory tests. Likewise, these indicators also have certain threshold points. Just as any disease can progress, so can the intensity of an indicator. But sometimes an indicator can be mild and remain mild indefinitely in the same way some illnesses don't progress. Other times, an indicator can start as mild and then become more severe, or it can start as intense or severe right away. Much depends on the nature of the health imbalance and the person. I know where these threshold points are in terms of their visibility from my many years of observation, but again, it's all subjective. It's my call, based on my personal decisions about their intensity."

"Did you say threshold *points*? There is more than one?"

"Well, now that you mention it, there is more than one."

"Let's distinguish as much as we can about your intensity perceptions."

"We already know there is a wide range of possible health imbalances for any body organ—asthma and lung cancer are not the same thing. But I am also talking about the range within the appearance of the respiratory indicator. Just as there is a physiological difference between lung cancer and asthma, there is also an indicator difference. The more intense the indicator appears to me, the more aggressive and life threatening the illness is. It's really pretty simple."

"It's possible that your perceptions are much more sensitive than conventional testing. That's how you pick up on health imbalances before a laboratory tests does. You aren't 'seeing' into the future. Instead, a possible explanation for your predictions coming true is that you have a more precise, more sensitive microscope than conventional medicine does."

"That brings up another important point, Beth. Since we are in the formative stages of the clinical use of indicators, do we want to condition my perceptions to duplicate what a conventional medical assessment can detect? If we continue to call my assessments as misses when the patient reports pain or symptoms, then are we conditioning my observations to detect less? Don't we want to allow this kind of perception to become an assessment style all its own? Keep in mind that statistically speaking, standard conventional medical tests, on average, have a margin for error or sometimes produce false positives. Do we want to consciously include an inherent level of error into my way of measuring health, or shall we let the body's language of health determine its own level of accuracy based on its own performance, not by comparison?"

"Since we already know the indicators can detect health imbalances in advance, let's consider that we need to be flexible if we want to learn more about how you perceive. We can satisfy these questions by creating a format that will not change the study protocol and will also allow for the assessment of varying intensities. There must be a conventional diagnosis established in order for you to register a hit. Yet we can make a note of the occurrences when you perceive an imbalance, the patient reports symptoms or discomfort, and conventional tests do not detect any imbalance. Obviously, a major benefit from these clinical trials would be to create a process for evaluating health conditions in advance. Besides, one purpose of the study is to measure the level of your perceptions. If you can identify health imbalances in the future, then it needs to be noted even if aside from the study. Let's also place emphasis on the intensity of the imbalances you can detect so we can build a system of threshold categories."

§ § §

One of the challenges I noted earlier is the slow progress of acceptance in our culture when it comes to the full use of the senses. To date, the lack of a generally accepted vocabulary to describe or explain nonordinary uses of the senses has offset the potency that our natural abilities have to offer. While there may be some jargon surrounding the phenomena, such as "Can you *feel* the energy in the room?" or "Your energy is *off* today," these expressions offer no value in the domain of science, especially in the arena of health care since medicine relies on facts, figures, and objectively measurable data.

As our sessions continued, the examination of patients provided us with more information to fill some of the gaps in our nonordinary vocabulary. The duration of our debriefing sessions lasted longer as Beth and I discussed many different ways to remove not only my own limits but the limits of anyone's perception. Beth showed me how open-minded a professional health care provider can be, and her knowledge of health and medicine brought new meaning to many of my uncertain perceptions. She explained to me that during her training as a nurse, it was not uncommon to spend a short period of time with a patient and know the status of a patient's health condition before any test results had returned with a diagnosis. In fact, my suspicions of others being able to see health imbalances were slowly solidifying; nurses knew how to perceive their patient's health. They only lacked a vocabulary that told them *how* they knew.

§ § §

Satisfied with my level of accuracy thus far in the clinical trials, I began working with clients outside the study. Many of the people who came to see me had unresolved health imbalances that conventional medicine could not identify, explain, or correct. While the study had prepared me for patients sitting silent before me as I gathered information, private sessions with clients were much more talkative, which was also a new experience for me. During these sessions, I heard about the many conventional medical practices explored by clients without proper identification of their elusive health problems.

Because the sessions were talkative, I could elaborate and provide all the detailed information that was available. I worked with people who had vaguely defined diagnoses or mysterious ailments. Although people often came to me with one particular health concern, I felt it was my responsibility to inform them of *all* the imbalances I perceived. The ninety minute sessions were paced to perform an entire body organ/system indicator analysis. I knew that this kind of comprehensive review could identify the sources of any imbalances and also give advance notice before any body organs or systems demonstrated signs of distress. People could then move quickly with their physicians to correct their health imbalances. I also worked with a few people who did not have any health concerns at the time but wanted to peek around the curtain and see what the future might hold; they wanted an indicator check-up.

I was surprised to learn how many people were experiencing confusion in the health care delivery system. They had already been to several physicians, yet their health imbalances remained undiagnosed, which meant they were improperly or ineffectively treated. The delay in accurate diagnosis had left people to wallow in physical pain and misery. During the course of these sessions, the combination of indicator data and discussions with the client about their health history and lifestyle allowed the client and me to derive a comprehensive plan to pursue with their physician. It was gratifying to me that the indicator assessments were of service to those who experienced confusion about the sources of their health imbalances.

However, it was frustrating for some of the people I counseled because their health care provider was unwilling to pursue any diagnostic investigations or treatments. Furthermore, if they told their physician that their health leads came from a "perceptive person," their physician would not take their examination requests seriously. But if people were not receiving medical support, follow-up treatment, and answers from their own physicians, how much benefit was truly achieved as a result of these private sessions? I began to rethink if this was the most effective venue to deliver this kind of information. When people returned to me and said their physician was unwilling to pursue their medical concerns, at least I had an alternative resource to offer. I referred them to Len and Beth's Bethesda medical practice since they were health care providers who would listen to patient concerns and take positive action.

However, in their quests for healing, people had growing expectations about what a meeting with me would produce. At first, they wanted an indicators assessment, but now they were asking me to perform health *corrections*. Their requests were not unreasonable. All they really wanted was to be well.

While I was confident about my abilities to *perceive* activity in the body through the indicators, *my perception or clinical demonstrations do not include diagnosing, influencing, alleviating, treating, or curing a disease in any way.* This presented me with a new set of challenges and an ethical dilemma. How does healing actually take place? Who actually performs the healing when someone is healed? Is it the practitioner who performs the healing, or is it the patient that allows healing to occur? Is the practitioner a conduit of healing or is the patient, or both? On a personal level, how could I affect a person's health during a ninety-minute meeting if their body and thought atmosphere were already prone to debilitation? It would be the same as putting air into a tire that has a leak in it. It might hold air temporarily, but sooner or later, the air would escape once more. I went in circles with these kinds of questions, and it all came back to the same place: Am I to become responsible for the content of the thought atmospheres of others and subsequently their health? I was simply reporting my observations; I was just the messenger.

Many people believe someone else has the power to heal them. They do not see how they are equal to the task. I wanted to empower people to reclaim and sustain their own health as a result of the sessions and information that their body brought forth. They wanted me to correct their health imbalances. I wanted them to understand that I can read from the book of their life, but I cannot write in the book of their life and restore their health. Only *they* can write in the book of their own life. We had arrived at a conflict of interest, and I did not know how to proceed.

Prominent Points for Chapter Review

- The body speaks its own language of health. Conventional medicine speaks the scientific language of health. Similarities and inconsistencies exist between these two languages.

- The body's response to injury or illness extends beyond pain or symptoms. The body also has an inherent ability to voice the response via the indicators.

- A one-to-one correlation has not been established between lifestyles and disease by medical science. The indicators track health changes based upon lifestyle choices for each individual.

- The threat to health reaches a certain threshold in order to cause an indicator to be present.

- Indicators can be present before conventional medical methods can detect any irregularities.

- Indicators have intensities.

- Allow for the body's logic. The body's perspective does not always equal the kind of rational format we would expect.

CHAPTER FOUR

Multiple Sclerosis or Misdiagnosis?

WHEN PEOPLE SEEK conventional health care, they are aware that a discovery process will occur, but they expect their health ailment to be diagnosed and treated within a reasonable amount of time. The discovery process can include tests, a period of waiting for test results, an assessment of those results, and a return visit to the physician's office to discuss the results. Pending the need for a referral to a medical specialist, a health recovery plan is usually created, which can include medications, diet changes or supplements, physical therapies, surgeries, or any combination thereof. However, some recovery plans can require secondary tests before treatments can begin. The desired end result, or cure, does not usually occur within a few hours or days. Inaccurate diagnosis and ineffective treatment plans can start the process of testing and waiting all over again in order to establish a recovery plan. Sometimes these health recovery plans work, and sometimes they do not.

A health assessment through body indicators is also a discovery process, but it is not a panacea and certainly not all knowing. Expectations and requests for health corrections became more frequent as I continued to work with people. I told Beth what was happening, and she understood my concerns, noting how frustrating it can be for both the patient and the health care practitioner if conventional treatment is not correcting the health imbalance. We both agreed that the best approach to supporting people was to learn as much as we could about the indicators. Since the clinical trials had provided us with answers to many of our questions thus far, we kept our focus to the study.

At this point, Beth and I had some ideas about how to concretize my indicator vocabulary. In order to make this technique accessible to others, we needed a common point of reference; we needed a common language. She suggested that we pause to establish the threshold criteria for the indicators before we assessed any more patients. The creation of these categories would allow us to identify and track health imbalances more clearly. There was much to consider in designing comprehensive categorical descriptions for the intensity levels of the indicators. We had to make sure the categories were precise so they would remain consistent over time. We finally arrived at taxonomy already familiar to conventional medicine, similar to the way a physician classifies a burn—by degrees. The following categories describe the intensity of indicators and the condition of health.

Body Organ/System Indicator Intensity Scale

First Degree:

- conventional medical exam may or may not reveal imbalance
- often chronic and mild in nature
- overall quality of life maintained
- can identify residual effects of system abnormalities now resolved
- can relate to an energetic that is not yet an issue in the physical plane
- quantitatively may represent 10-20 percent of a body system out of balance
- examples of first degree conditions are IBS, allergies, candida, high blood pressure, past surgeries, and residual health imbalances

Second Degree:

- conventional medical exam will most likely reveal imbalance
- often chronic and possibly advancing in presence
- overall quality of life may or may not be affected
- threat to the body system greater than first degree
- illness can be competing for dominion over body's natural balance
- quantitatively may represent 20-40 percent of a body system out of balance
- examples of second degree conditions are cysts, tumors (benign or malignant), and heart disease

Third Degree:

- conventional medical exam will most likely reveal imbalance
- often chronic and severe in nature

- overall quality of life is affected
- body system is completely out of balance—the illness dominates
- quantitatively may represent > 50 percent of a body system out of balance
- examples of third degree conditions are invasive metastasizing growths, cardiac arrest, or any health condition that causes death

With the intensity categories defined, the clinical study resumed and the indicator health assessments were reported in the following manner.

Patient 01007: "Jerry"

John: This patient has a second-degree genital/urinary indicator, a first-degree blood indicator that correlates to high blood pressure, a first-degree spinal indicator, a first-degree eye indicator, a second-degree cardiovascular indicator, and a first-degree digestive indicator.

Beth: The conventional diagnoses include enlarged prostate, a history of sexually transmitted disease, high blood pressure, degenerative disc disease, chronic back pain, and had vision correction surgery, but there is no record of any gastrointestinal or cardiovascular problems.

John: The digestive indicator is mild, so it may not show up on a conventional test. The cardiovascular is pretty obvious though.

Beth: Well, the only possible connection that I can make is that the patient is a long-term smoker, and that might have an effect on his cardiovascular system.

John: The tobacco use is taking its toll. The cardiovascular system is indicating that the tobacco use could become more of an issue in the future. But there is something else that concerns me.

Beth: What's that?

John: Well, I didn't want to say anything in front of the gentleman. I figured I would wait until you and I were alone because I am not sure about what I saw. Plus, it will sound absolutely ridiculous, and I don't want to reduce my accuracy score by what seems bizarre to me.

Beth: Just tell me what you see.

John: Well, I see a breast indicator.

Beth: Okay . . .

John: Well, I have only seen a breast indicator in women. This patient is a man, and he has a female breast indicator. It is obvious. I have never seen a man with a breast indicator, and I don't know what to make of this.

Beth: That's because he has been diagnosed with—

Just then the door knob turned, and Dr. Wisneski walked into the room and sat down with a thick folder in his hand.

Len: Good morning, you two. I thought I would stop in for a moment. I have been looking over the reports from the study, and this is seminal work, very impressive.

Beth and I shared with Len more of the study results and the newly defined categories. We also told him about how we conducted our debriefings, and some of the questions we still had about comparing the indicators with the conventional assessments. But I took advantage of Len's unexpected visit.

John: Since you are here, Len, maybe you can make some sense out of this for me. We were talking about a patient I just saw. The patient is male and has a female breast indicator. The breast indicator is clear as day, but . . . he's a guy.

Len: Which patient are we talking about?

Beth told Len the patient's name.

Len: That's because he has gynecomastia.

John: What's that?

Len: It's a condition of breast enlargement that sometimes happens to men as a side effect of certain high blood pressure medications.

John: He didn't appear to have enlarged breasts. I have never heard of such a thing, but I wasn't going to say anything about it.

Beth gave me an odd glance before she spoke again.

Beth: It's really important that you don't analyze or doubt your perceptions. You need to trust your awareness and report *whatever* information you receive. Otherwise, you are filtering the information with your expectations, and you will end up skewing the results.

I was not over intellectualizing or doubting my perceptions, but I was not telling Len and Beth everything either. Unknown to them, I was holding back information. Of course, I wanted to get the best possible performance rating, but I had to maintain their confidence with the study and with me. If I told them *everything*, it might sound too weird for any scientific basis. Even though we had already accomplished much, I was not sure how this information related to the study. I was not going to say anything until I knew exactly what it meant—until the moment was right.

Patient 02008: "Helen"

John: The patient has a first-degree respiratory indicator, a second-degree digestive indicator—it looks like IBS, but there is another digestive aspect present that might progress. There is a second-degree spinal indicator, a first-degree breast indicator showing past activity, a first-degree reproductive indicator relating to infertility, and a thyroid indicator, but for some reason, I cannot assign a degree to it. I don't think I have ever seen a thyroid indicator like this. There is something unique about it. The indicator is telling me that the thyroid condition is present but also not present at the same time. Something has been done to correct it. I'll take another chance with reducing my accuracy, and so I won't withdraw my thyroid indicator.

Beth: The patient has a history of tobacco abuse, has IBS, and a history of Hepatitis B. There is degenerative disc disease and a history of a motor vehicle accident, which caused damage to the spine. There is a history of a nonmalignant breast tumor and a history of hypothyroidism. But what is unique is that she has been hypothyroid since birth. There is no medical evidence of infertility.

John: Does she have children?

Beth: No.

John: I have more information about her thyroid. Tell me, does she suffer from any symptoms or discomfort from her hypothyroidism?

Beth: No.

John: What is her age?

Beth: She's forty-seven.

John: Because there is something unique about her thyroid indicator, somehow her thyroid has adapted to this hypofunctioning condition during the course of her lifetime. Her body has adjusted to the extent that it is now considered to be a normal condition to her whole body system, which is why she does not experience any discomfort or symptoms. Her indicator has altered its appearance to reflect this adaptation. Beth, a thought has just occurred to me. Could it be possible to treat the indicators?

Beth: What do you mean?

John: Let's look at this from another perspective. Do people have an indicator because they have a health imbalance, or do they have a health imbalance because they have an indicator? I am asking which comes first, the chicken or the egg? Since we have already noticed indicators before any signs, symptoms, or tests can detect any imbalance, is it possible that the indicators bring forth other messages that we do not know how to read yet? The indicators aren't the cause of disease, but if they are some kind of precursor to illness, maybe we could learn how to reduce the intensity of indicators and, therefore, reduce the pain, discomfort, or symptoms of the illness. Better yet, Beth, what would it take to remove an indicator and avert illness altogether?

Beth: Those are some really great questions. It's possible that the indicators hold clues to how disease develops in the human body. They might even help us redefine and redirect some of our conventional approaches to health and healing. We'll have to talk more about this later. The next patient is here. I will show her in.

Our meetings at Wyngate Medical Park turned into discussions about how to integrate indicators into the health care delivery system. Indicators could assist health care providers to better diagnose medical conditions and perhaps steer the body toward healing and wellness. We wanted to know how to affect the indicators, and if so, would it cause any measurable change in a health imbalance or laboratory tests? We also wondered further if the indicators could be used as a basis for new clinical therapies.

§ § §

I continued to work with people outside of the study. I kept Beth advised of my progress and what I was learning about people, health, and indicators. By now, my health assessments had become routine. I approached my sessions with clients with the same protocol as the clinical study. I told people to not disclose their health histories or any health complaints until after I had rendered my assessment. At the completion of our session, people had useful information that they could bring to their health care provider for follow-up tests and treatment. But the conversations kept coming back to the fact that people did not want more tests. They wanted healing. The amount of frustration I encountered from people during sessions increased. *Something* needed to happen soon in the way that I worked with people to support their healing, and that *something* was just around the corner.

One day a woman named Rhonda called me. I was about to explain the session protocol to her, but before I could stop her from telling me anything about her health, she verbally splattered me with all of her peculiar symptoms. She also enumerated the endless list of conventional tests she had already been through. Yet her health imbalance remained a complete mystery to her and her doctors. She experienced various and seemingly unrelated symptoms: severe headaches, changes in skin texture in her abdominal region, vision problems with severe pain and loss of muscle control in her right eye, and vertigo. She was under the care of a neurologist, ophthalmologist, and general practitioner, and all conventional medical tests to date were inconclusive.

In addition, the months of emotional and psychological stress from the unresolved medical problems had taken their toll. Rhonda was at her wits' end; she was drowning in the deep waters of her symptoms and needed to get out fast.

We met, and I performed an indicator assessment and reviewed all of her body organs and systems with her. Although she had neurological symptoms, she did not demonstrate a neurological indicator. Although she had skin texture changes, I did not perceive an imbalance in her skin. She had a very mild eye indicator, in the first-degree, but certainly not prevalent enough to explain why she had lost control of her eye muscles or experienced such severe pain. The eye indicator may have been present because her eyes were somehow affected by her health imbalance, but the low intensity level of the indicator suggested there was no pathology or actual illness of the eyes. However, she had a prominent thyroid indicator. I recommended that she return to her physicians with this information for their immediate evaluation, and she agreed.

Her next doctor appointment was with her ophthalmologist, and she asked me to accompany her to the office. She said there were times when the ophthalmologist performed treatments that would cause her eyes to become very sensitive to light, and operating a motor vehicle after her appointment was very dangerous. She asked me to drive her to and from her appointment, and I accepted. Since I had escorted her to the office, she decided to take it one step further and insisted I be present in the examination room while the ophthalmologist administered treatment. I was introduced to her physician as a friend who drove her to the office and nothing more. However, Rhonda was not one to mince words. Once the three of us were in the examination room, she wanted to know if the indicator information was correct. She asked the ophthalmologist several questions and wanted to know if her thyroid could be the cause of the loss of eye muscle control and affect her vision. The ophthalmologist immediately dismissed her thyroid as a possible cause of her condition—end of discussion.

I was between a doc and a hard place. Rhonda looked at me as if to say, "You're fired." I did not feel it was appropriate to challenge the physician in his own office, nor was that the purpose of my visit. Since I could not reveal the indicator content of our session, I remained silent and bit my tongue all the while. The drive home gave Rhonda and me an opportunity to talk more about our session, but it brought her no comfort. Since her ophthalmologist had dismissed the thyroid, she dismissed the indicator information she received from me. She was deeply disenchanted. I, on the other hand, was not going to allow the information to be discarded so easily since Rhonda had an obvious thyroid indicator. I had already been through this once before with the woman in Len's office. I was committed to bringing benefit and resolution to Rhonda's health crisis, and I remained in contact with her after the visit to the ophthalmologist.

Her mysterious symptoms persisted and intensified. Each time we spoke on the telephone, she was increasingly despondent. She found it difficult to focus on the day's events or menial tasks. She could no longer engage in activities that brought her pleasure such as reading a book without enduring pain. The most detrimental of all was living in confusion and not knowing what was happening while her health decayed with each passing day. Since all of her medical tests had been inconclusive, and based on her symptoms, her physicians prepared Rhonda for the worst—a diagnosis of multiple sclerosis (MS). She notified me to say she was to meet with her physicians to begin MS testing procedures and wanted to know why I did not mention MS during our session. I told her that she did not demonstrate the kind of indicator I have seen with people who have MS. I asked her if there was any way that her thyroid could be reevaluated before they began the tests. But she was not confident with my assessments, and with nowhere else to turn, Rhonda followed the instructions of her physicians and began the testing procedures for diagnosing MS.

After preliminary MS laboratory tests returned negative results, Rhonda was hopeful, but her physicians were not pacified. They remained *certain* that she had MS and told her so. When Rhonda informed me that she had been scheduled for a spinal tap, I emphasized that her previous tests for MS had returned negative results. Once again, I suggested that Rhonda insist that her physicians reexamine her thyroid; it certainly would not be as expensive or as painful as a spinal tap. For whatever reasons, her physicians were not willing to include Rhonda in the decision-making process about her own health and would not reevaluate her thyroid. I could not understand why this inquiry about her thyroid was causing such resistance from her physicians.

Once Rhonda recovered from the spinal tap, she contacted me to tell me that her test results had returned negative; she did not have MS. This was both the good news and the bad news. It was a relief to her and her family that her tests returned negative, but she was right back to where she started with no clear answers. Several months passed, and Rhonda remained in limbo about her health while her symptoms persisted. Rhonda continued to bounce from physician to physician until she eventually ended up at an internist. When the internist requested and reviewed Rhonda's health history, the blood panel from earlier in the previous year clearly identified that Rhonda's thyroid was in a "hyper" range condition. She asked Rhonda if she had been informed of this, but it had gone overlooked by *all* of her physicians—a neurologist, ophthalmologist, and general practitioner. The internist recommended Rhonda have her thyroid checked again, and when she did, Rhonda was formally diagnosed with Grave's disease (a hyperthyroid condition and the root cause of all her seemingly unrelated symptoms).

Finally, Rhonda had the crucial information she had been seeking—an *accurate* medical diagnosis. Now she could build her recovery plan to restore her health and return to vitality. Although the biological source of her illness was confirmed, her journey of recovery had only begun. Her physicians recommended that her thyroid be surgically removed or radioactively killed, and she would have to live the rest of her life on chemical additives. This did not appeal to her in the least. Since the indicator assessment turned out to be accurate after all, she was eager to resume meetings with me. We discussed her concerns, and she affirmed that her body's natural choice was to remain intact and fully functional.

At this point, the answers were coming much easier to Rhonda. Her search for a physician who would include her in the decision-making process was brief. Given that Rhonda's condition required an endocrinologist, a physician that specialized in thyroid imbalances, it all came together effortlessly. The supervising physician of the clinical study, Dr. Leonard Wisneski, was the logical choice to establish a health recovery plan for Rhonda. She met with Dr. Wisneski, and she was delighted to find that he was also a proponent of restoring her thyroid to its normal range of function. The idea of removing or rendering it permanently disabled and Rhonda living on medications for the rest of her life did not appeal to him either.

As the first step in recovery, Rhonda was placed on medications that would support her thyroid function. Dr. Wisneski began a process of balancing medications to achieve the proper dosage, which was a normal procedure for her hyperthyroid condition. However, Rhonda was anxious to get back to her usual self and was not interested in waiting for positive results. She had waited long enough, and she wanted to know *now* if the treatments were going to be effective. Her level of energy remained low, and she returned to the Bethesda office at regular intervals for blood tests to measure progress. Although her test did not show any progress, she responsibly continued to meet with Dr. Wisneski for treatment. He reassured her that it was not unusual for a period of time to pass before her thyroid would respond to treatment, especially while he was seeking the precise blend of medications to properly rebalance her thyroid function. Rhonda and I remained in contact, and I continued to look for any opportunity to reveal more information about her thyroid.

I recalled earlier in the clinical study when I observed the woman whose thyroid had been in a hypo state since birth. I was able to see via her indicator that her thyroid had *already* compensated for the imbalance. I had observed her thyroid *after* the period of being reregulated. I wondered if it was possible to observe changes in an indicator *while* the body was in the process of reregulating—in other words, healing. Could an indicator communicate when and if the body organ or system was moving toward wholeness and health? I had to find out. Since Rhonda's thyroid was in a state of decompensation, watching her thyroid indicator during the process of treatment provided me with a unique situation.

Rhonda continued to meet with me for follow up observations. Unfortunately, there was no observable change in her thyroid indicator, as she lingered in lethargy and her symptoms persisted. While Dr. Wisneski reevaluated her mix of medications, I reevaluated my perceptions. The information that I had kept from Len and Beth was beginning to make sense to me now but I was dealing with raw perceptual data that required more translation. Rhonda's body was saying *something* else, but I could not put my finger on it. On a very basic level of understanding, Rhonda's thyroid was "misbehaving" at the expense of the rest of her body system, but why?

I was also realizing that the indicators were telling me illness is more than a body organ or system going out of balance. If our psychological studies maintain that human behavior is motivated, then by extension, the same could apply to the behavior of disease within the human body. But what would motivate a particular body organ or system to behave inconsistently with the body's natural harmony? If motivations are not random, as psychological studies also maintain, then body organ or system irregularities could be motivated by the same or equal reasons for anyone who experiences that particular body organ or system irregularity. For example, people who have a thyroid imbalance may also have a consistent theme or message that their body is communicating to them and causing their thyroid to activate. It was time to get back to basics and comprehend the indicators at the fundamental level.

I had to go beneath the surface of what I could see. By describing the characteristics of the indicators, I might receive more information about exactly what the body is projecting. In this example, I explored the thyroid indicator, and my findings produced the following:

Thyroid Indicator

- One does not look at the throat region where the thyroid resides to detect the indicator.
- The area of the body where the indicator projects from is the cheeks of the face.
- The indicator is symbolized by holes in the cheeks, much the same as a sponge in your kitchen sink.
- To perceive the indicator, you "feel" the holes under the surface of the skin as you look at the cheeks, but you will not see holes.
- The larger, more concentrated, and more area of the cheeks the holes cover, the more intense the thyroid imbalance.

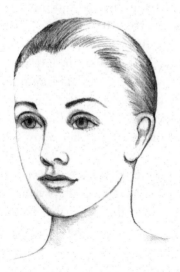

Without Indicator

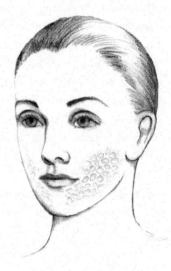

Thyroid Indicator

As I stared at my illustration, I was drawn to the fundamental significance of the holes. I was curious to know if a metaphoric interpretation existed. The relevance of this particular indicator depicted by holes and a thyroid imbalance might have something in common, I thought. Since the language of indicators is like a child, I looked at the indicator through the eyes of a child once more. The thyroid indicator is full of holes as though the cheeks have been perforated. It brought to mind for me a colander for pasta; it does not hold water—it permits the water to pass through. Therefore, I arrived at a most crude interpretation. The thyroid indicator holes represent the inability to hold or retain fluidity or content. The holes allow some kind of seepage, perhaps something that would normally not leak through. A healthy thyroid would retain what an unhealthy thyroid loses, thus representing the loss of something that needs to be restored, but what?

The physiological function of the thyroid is to secrete hormones that regulate metabolism—the conversion of oxygen and calories into energy. The other body organs rely on the proper function of this conversion process; it is essential for the success of the whole body system. When the thyroid moves into a hypo (too slow) or hyper (too fast) state, the latter being the case with Rhonda, then its performance is unnatural to sustain the normal functions of the body. A thyroid out of balance can wreak all kinds of havoc on the body system accompanied by any number of mysterious physical signs and symptoms.

This conversion process of oxygen and calories is what provides the body with energy; therefore, we are talking about the regulation of the body's metabolic power production and supply. Since we are examining the process of energy conversion, let us convert the metabolic into the metaphoric. What if this disruption to Rhonda's metabolic power supply equates to a metaphor that means Rhonda is also experiencing a disruption to her "personal power" supply? Could it be that her thyroid has mimicked the way that Rhonda positions herself in her relationships, an internal demonstration of the external dynamics of her life?

I contacted Rhonda to ask if my ideas held any resonance for her. I invited her to look for areas in her life where she might be giving her personal power away to others or to circumstances. Awareness is the first step toward reclaiming health, but for Rhonda, that meant moving into areas of personal discomfort and challenging certain relationships in order to reclaim her personal power. However, since she was consumed by the collective debilitating physiological effects of a thyroid gone wild, she could not focus on anything beyond her physical distress. She needed to stop the bleeding, so to speak, before she could address her personal relationships.

Rhonda and I met again a few months later to reevaluate her thyroid indicator. This time, as I watched her approach and before she said hello to me, I immediately noticed her indicator had changed. It had reduced its intensity and was moving toward complete absence; the holes were filling in. I told her what I saw and that it looked as though her body was responding to the most recent treatment Dr. Wisneski had administered. She told me she was feeling like her "old self" again and that Dr. Wisneski had made some adjustments to her medications and dosage within the last seventy-two hours. Shortly thereafter, Rhonda had blood drawn and a panel performed. The medical test confirmed that her thyroid was returning to the normal range.

Rhonda was elated! This was also exciting news for her family. By balancing her system with the appropriate combinations of medication, she was no longer consumed by her overwhelming symptoms. Rhonda had been pulled from the deep end of the pool, but she was not out of the water yet. In the shallow end, she could breathe the air once more, and now she could focus on the nonphysiological matter at hand—the interruption of her personal power. Rhonda met with Beth for Gestalt therapy sessions and also a bonding psychotherapist to challenge her self-defeating patterns in her personal relationships. After two years of working with these collected aspects of both her thyroid and personal power, Rhonda's thyroid has returned to and remained in complete health. She no longer takes medication, beta blockers, herbs, or additives of any kind. Rhonda was grateful for Dr. Wisneski's sensitivity to her needs and for taking a healing path that allowed her to keep her thyroid intact. The long period of living in confusion and disarray with mounting medical expenses had finally come to an end.

I did not have my hands around *all* the answers, but it was becoming abundantly clear that revealing the meaning or message behind any health imbalance most likely requires a committed and perhaps rigorous self-discovery process. Even though the imbalances in our health are not based solely on cause and effect, we unconsciously organize the content of the thought atmosphere, and ultimately, that content is manifested in the body. Since deciphering the messages from the core of our being is a subjective process, if we do not receive the messages or interpret them accurately, the body does not remain idle. The metabolic stage is set for disease, and the countdown to illness begins.

However, I approached my sessions with a certain level of passive politeness. Once I identified distressed body organs or systems, I invited people to survey their lives and look for limiting content in their thought atmosphere. I assumed that since people stated they were genuinely interested in reclaiming their health, they would be motivated to act by the information I shared with them. But the mere suggestion that they might be contributing to their own health problems was often met with deflection and denial. When clients assured me there was no limiting content in their lives *and everything was just wonderful,* I had graciously acquiesced. However, I found myself discarding information of Gibraltar proportions during these sessions simply because the client said that what I told them "could not be true."

§ § §

By and large, people seek a life of comfort. Or perhaps a more accurate statement is that people seek a life defined and contained within a certain kind of comfort zone. This zone includes vast areas of psychological and emotional ease, in addition to the basics of requirements of food, shelter, and so on. There are many who will remain safely within the perimeter of their comfort zone throughout a lifetime. But comfort can also mean becoming content with self-defeating behaviors that operate in our lives every day, either consciously or unconsciously. Not everyone has a desire to live a self-examined life or cast light on the shadows of their thought atmosphere or behaviors. Subsequently, revealing the sources of illness can be a threat to people's comfortable lives. But if remaining in our comfort zones provided the answers to life's mysteries of health and disease, we would already live in a society free of illness. Because our culture has trained us to maintain a personal comfort zone and avoid situations where we encounter conflict or discord, these keys to healing are seldom found. If the success to long-term health and wellness is to identify self-defeating thoughts and behaviors, then going boldly where we have never gone before becomes paramount.

People continued to meet with me to resolve their health problems and find healing. But in order to bring the foundation of their illness into the open meant leading people out of their comfort zone and into unknown territories. I had to reorganize the way I structured my sessions to remove these barriers to fostering health. After working with Rhonda, I revisited each of the indicators and found several other metaphors for the metabolic messages of the body.* The same way that I introduced Rhonda to her own power struggle, I presented this metaphoric information during sessions to support people's discovery process and their reclamation of health. Once again, the information was received about as well as a ketchup-and-honey sandwich. People contested the additional information that I brought forward during our sessions. Stoically, they insisted that they had no "issues" in their life to address. There were no self-defeating behaviors to be revealed in their relationships with others or with self. Yet the years of negativity and denial that had accumulated in their cell tissues remained while their body waited for them to heed the call. Their health imbalances did not develop overnight and probably were not going to vanish overnight, especially if they would not admit to possibly affecting their own thought atmosphere and, therefore, their health. However, they needed to know they could improve their health by challenging the intra-and interpersonal dynamics of their lives. Primarily, they needed to become aware that these dynamics existed before they could make any substantial changes. But it was not going to be easy to counsel people when their thought atmosphere contained huge amounts of resistance, and at the same time, they wanted instant health corrections.

Quite often, when people met with me, it was because conventional medical methods failed to resolve their health problems. Nothing is perfect in this world, whether it is a conventional medical assessments or otherwise. However, I no longer wondered why conventional methods were ineffective for some people because their obstinate positions would deflect even the most potent of conventional medical treatments or medications.

I thought that people would welcome the health information I had to offer, but I began to question their true desire to heal. Did they want to remain tied to the dramas that their health imbalances enabled rather than listen to their own body? I was just the messenger, but the messages were not getting through.

---

* These metabolic messages will be presented in the illustrations chapter.

Prominent Points of Chapter Review

- Indicators provide information beyond the existence or potential threat of a health imbalance.

- The indicators reflect the intensity and other qualitative characteristics of a health imbalance.

- Indicators are interactive. They respond by reducing their intensity and appearance when the body is receiving effective medications or treatments.

- Indicators can reveal the metaphoric motivations that set the stage for organ disease.

CHAPTER FIVE

Contrary Conditioning

I N THE MONTHS that passed, I refocused on our meetings in the Bethesda office. The research study had become an evolutionary process for Beth and me and our ideas about health came closer together. After Beth and I assessed patients and compared results, we let our minds roam and entertained new ideas about the directions of health care. Our own form of medical anthropology emerged as we searched the history of medicine for any mention of these indicators. If other medical practitioners had observed them over the centuries, we might be able to trace the lineage of the indicators to an origin. Beth was also curious to know if the model of indicators could be overlaid onto other medical traditions. She suspected that there might be some similarities found within other medical disciplines such as traditional Chinese medicine or the Indian chakra system. While other medical traditions had methods for identifying health imbalances, none of them referred to the indicators. However, we remained vigilant for any consistent elements that we might have overlooked. Even as we broadened our understanding, we continued to compare the indicators to other medical disciplines, conventional or otherwise. These discussions led to planning several other clinical project designs and new ways to test my sensory cursor. However, the answers that had come thus far, although meaningful, had only stimulated more complex questions. Foremost on our minds was exactly how this process of health detection and indicators actually worked and what *other* information the body had to offer.

The clinical study had also provided Beth with information that she had not anticipated; information we could not explain but also could not ignore. At this point, necessity expanded Beth's role in the study. The management of the protocol and grading my medical assessments were now only a portion of her supervisory duties. The needs of our research required her to move into a role of integrator between our research findings and conventional medical reasoning. We suspected that the indicators held several as yet undecipherable clues relating to health and disease.

But we were confronted by large amounts of raw perceptual data that required translation before we could set any theories in place. Whenever we sought the conventions of medicine to assist us with translation, we were consistently met by the empty pockets of Western science. There was simply no resource of information available as we continued to pick at the locks of health and disease by turning the tumblers of perception.

With conventional resources exhausted, we only had each other to look to for answers. Beth had asked me several times to search my past for clues, but it was my turn to inquire about her past. She had been met by several inconsistencies in the conventional medical community along her path of completing her degrees in nursing and professional development. She had questioned the fundamental structure of health care long ago because she felt that some of the conventional treatments offered fell short of the prescribed therapeutic goals of healing. These contraries became the genesis of her departure from a conventional medical practice. Eventually, her search compelled the reinvention of herself as an integrative nurse practitioner. By the time she began working with Len, her approach to health and healing was refreshing and astute. Most of all, she demonstrated a genuine commitment to the people she treated accompanied by a deep desire to empower the quality of health care she delivered every day.

Beth already recognized that a critical component of healing relied on revealing the underlying messages from the body to the patient. She found this communication loop was essential to her patients' recovery process. However, it was not always easy for the patient to embrace this connection and hear the underlying messages from within. She took it upon herself to facilitate this union of awareness and receptivity by bringing these personal elements to light in a way that was effectively received. Since our research study had filled in many of the holes that conventional medicine had not during her years of academia, she was anxious to apply the indicators in her own patient practice. We spoke regularly and called each other on the phone to share our latest "what if" sensory perception scenarios. Beth felt that if we could further describe and understand the constructs of the indicators, it would increase diagnostic proficiency, which was her primary objective as a health care provider. As a scientist, she needed to know exactly how these perceptions related to the course of conventional medical practices. Beth became the modem between the indicators and allopathic medicine.

We were motivated to combine our research with Beth's patient practice and clinically broaden the scope of health care delivery. However, given the scientifically sensitive subject matter under investigation, we needed a platform to present our ideas that were rational and accessible. Our next challenge was that the empirical evidence from our study had limited access if the ability to perceive indicators resided only with me. All along, I maintained that others use their senses in ways that closely resemble mine but it was time to find out. I was curious to know if others would describe the indicators in the same way as I or would they have their own particular idiom. We both knew that if we were going to capture the attention of the health care delivery system, we needed to demonstrate a coherent use of the senses and the indicators.

Aside from the clinical study, the course of our research incorporated the examination of perceptual commonalties among people and how lifestyle choices influence the function of our five physical sensory inputs.

During our meetings in the Bethesda office, we examined my own sensory development from birth to adulthood to create a perceptual template. Our conversations did not reveal any information to suggest that external factors were responsible for making these perceptions possible for me. Although there were a few external factors that we ruled out as responsible for my ability to detect indicators. For example, people often ask me if I have a special diet. All I can say is that some of my most accurate health assessments were conducted on days filled with pizza and doughnuts. I do not have a special diet; I eat and drink whatever I like. I have not had a near-death experience, nor was I struck by lightning as an origin for these perceptions. People often ask me if I meditate in order to perceive the body indicators. While I continue to explore the benefits of meditation, it has no observable effect on my abilities to perceive body indicators. This is not to negate that people can access enhanced states of awareness *during* or *after* meditation, but in my case, it does not apply to blending the senses. The health perceptions I make are available to me while I am walking down the street, talking on the telephone, playing a musical instrument, or operating a motor vehicle. In other words, the perception of indicators is possible while you are engaged in other activities; it is not a fragile state of perception.

However, what I have found to be most effective during my sensory development is the deliberate increase of my own situational awareness. What this means is that I have a practice of living my life from a self-examined position. This is much the same as having a personal observer or auditor of my behavioral patterns and interactions except in this case, the auditor is *me*. What this means is that I seek to be as present as possible to the life that I live. Our daily experience of life is much like operating a motor vehicle. When we drive down the road, we all have blind spots, areas in our periphery that we cannot see. I place my awareness on my unawareness so that I may increase my perceptual acuity and reduce the area of my blind spots. Participation in my own awareness can fluctuate on a moment-to-moment basis as a result of any number of distractions I may encounter every day. For that reason, I set an intention to increase my participation in my awareness every day, and some days are certainly more successful than others. Perhaps it is a form of active meditation but a practice nonetheless.

However, Beth was looking for a specific mechanism to explain my observations. Although we had done it many times before, retracing my footsteps from youth had not produced any pieces to the puzzle. But Beth was certain we had overlooked something that may have seemed inconsequential yet was probably an important clue. This time, she shifted her inquiries about my childhood experiences *before* I began noticing these indicators. She wanted to thoroughly examine the broad premise of my sensory development during the formative stages. Instead of looking for experiences unique to me, she purposely looked for experiences consistent to all people during youth.

To a child, the world is a theater of infinite dimension. Children are the open vessels of receptivity during their early years; they have not yet been told to place restrictions on their reality. They live without perceptual limits, and this curious freedom is extremely powerful. Left intact, healthy curiosity can produce a lifelong foundation of *sensitive* sensory proclivities. I shared with Beth some of the other kinds of perceptual experiences I had during youth. These experiences were not about indicators—they were about the atmosphere. At the time, I did not make the connection between the two. It never occurred to me that the indicators and the atmosphere formed a coalition of health.

During the summer months of youth, I visited my grandparents in Idaho. My grandfather was an avid fly fisherman, and he had a room in his basement dedicated to the sacred art of fly tying. It was a full-fledged sportsman shrine—special lighting, a squeaky swivel chair, a magnifying glass the size of a dinner plate, and an enormous collection of animal pelts and fur stored in a large library card catalogue cabinet to hold them all.

The fly-tying room was my grandfather's hallowed sanctuary, a place he relished unto himself. I was only allowed to enter under his supervision, which was rare, and in his absence the door was tightly locked. The mystique made the desire to get inside all the more tempting, and there were times that I would sneak downstairs to check the lock just to be sure. On one occasion, the knob turned and clicked, the door opened, and I found myself standing alone in grandfather's chamber of secrets. I was proud of my success, and as I cherished the moment of breeching the forbidden threshold, something else caught my attention. Even though I stood there alone, it felt as though my grandfather was in the room with me. Or perhaps a more accurate description is that I could feel my grandfather's presence even in his absence. His essence hung as if dust in the air, a soft floating imprint of his identity upon the atmosphere. It is important to note that I did not see anything floating in the air. In fact, there was nothing additional in my field of view aside from a room with old furniture and fly-tying equipment. But I had to know what this feeling meant, what was happening. And so I allowed myself to be completely enveloped by these stimulations in the air.

I noticed that if I closed my eyes, I did not feel his presence as strongly; there was a slight disconnection. I realized how much the visual component of this experience linked me to the unseen feeling qualities in the atmosphere. The longer I spent with this visual kinesthetic experience, the more information came forward, and the atmosphere seemed to hold information about my grandfather's personality, about his emotions.

Suddenly, a noise came from outside the door. My grandfather came in and I had been found out. As he entered the room, it became apparent to me that there were now two versions of his presence to notice—his actual physical presence and his presence that was held in the atmosphere. The two became one when he stepped into the room, as if a hand was sliding into a glove. His actual personal presence matched the sensations that I perceived in the atmosphere. I was fascinated by this atmospheric activity, and I sought opportunities to repeat the experience wherever I went.

Perhaps you can recall visiting a relative or friend and having a similar experience. It may have been a garage, sewing room, or kitchen where the person spent a great deal of time. Or instead of a room, it may have been a favorite chair, a dress, a jewelry box, or any other personal item of significance that allowed you to perceive their presence. On the other hand, your perception may have seemed more general to you. You may have noticed qualities in their entire household atmosphere that were simply different from your home. Their house may have seemed more peaceful, tranquil, happier, or even safer than your own. Or perhaps you noticed these sensations but never lent them much attention because there were no words to describe it. But one thing was for sure—it did not *feel* the same as your own home.

The years of our youth held profound experiences, both significant and subtle, that we could not explain largely because we lacked a vocabulary to describe the territory that exists beyond the fringes of five sensory perceptions. Young people often look to their parents or the adult culture for answers and understanding. Since the adult community often clings to standardized thoughts, children generally do not receive the affirmation or explanations they require to hone the skills that emerge naturally and give meaning to these free-form sensory experiences. It is only a matter of time until limits are placed on a child's perceptual individuality and the innate expansion of their sensory frontiers.

An excellent example of this perceptual pruning was shared with me while I was leading a seminar. A gentleman attending the program shared his experience of working with "youth at risk" in the Bronx. He told me that during early development, children will regularly demonstrate their perceptual freedoms. When children are in grammar school and the teacher holds a quarter in his or her hand and shows it to the class with the instruction to "draw this," children respond most creatively. He observed how several children drew the teacher's hand holding the quarter with intricate anatomical detail resembling childlike works of Leonardo Da Vinci. Some drew the architecture of the quarter depicting each metallic ridge cut on the coin's circumference and the portrait profile of President George Washington. Other children drew the entire scene; the teacher standing before the class with the coin in hand, what was written on the blackboard behind the teacher, the clock on the wall showing the time of day, and so on. He noted that each child had their own perceptual reality. Every picture drawn was a unique reflection of how each child constructs their perception; no two drawings were alike. However, by the end of grammar school, when faced with the same instructional task by the teacher to draw the quarter, all the children in the classroom drew only the quarter.

While this example of perceptual pruning may seem insignificant, or perhaps even necessary to a standardized society, the developmental shifts are conditionally devastating. I am not the first to suggest that our culture is based in intellectual prejudice and censorship, but if our system of education narrows the ordinary uses of the senses, then what chance do *nonordinary* uses possibly have to develop? As children grow, intellectual obedience comes early with the dawn of perceptual rules. Without a support structure, an individual child would have to make a concerted effort, often in the face of adversity, to nurture their aspiring perceptions. Eventually, children arrive at a choice point between the natural perceptual abilites they possess and the intellectual insistence of the collective culture—the road *most* traveled. This is only one in a series of road splits that children encounter on the journey to adulthood. The sensory splits occur gradually and cumulatively that each individual episode of the limiting effects seldom becomes apparent until much later. By the time most children arrive in their early twenties, many of their perceptual capacities lay in fragments. Since uncommon perceptions have no place in an adult reality of conformity, the daily expectations of completing tasks are easiest met by surrendering to a standardized world of logic, reason, and measurable performance.

I avoided as many sensory splits as possible during my youth. Even though I openly accepted the world of logic and reason that was presented by society at large, I quietly cultivated my perceptual flexibility. It was not because I knew better, but because my perceptions were reinforced by the feedback I received about people's health. I knew that what I was seeing was natural and *factual*, not fantasy, and so I learned to live with one foot on the brake of conformity and the other on the throttle of expansion.

Later on, it occurred to me that there are common circumstances in every adult's life where subtle expansions of perception are often exercised. It seems that the perceptual freedoms of childhood are never lost; they are merely frozen in the winters of your past. These circumstances are not generally discussed openly, and the lack of vocabulary, among other reasons, prevents validation, but they do exist. I believe that once you learn to recognize these experiences and affirm them in your conscious mind, this will become clear. Search yourself, and you will find that the icicles of perception drip from the warm roof of recollection every day. If you stand still and stretch out your hands, you can catch the warm drops of sensitivity once again. But do not just touch them *you must feel them.*

Recall a time when you were at home *and alone.* Notice your level of activity and notice that whether you are at still point, such as reading a book, or at power point, such as running on the treadmill, the atmosphere of your living space is influenced by this activity. In between still point and power point is a gradient range of activities such as listening to music, watching television, cooking in the kitchen, and so on. The degree of your physical activity stimulates the local atmosphere in ways that you are normally accustomed to and there is nothing unusual to notice.

However, while your physical activities are obvious, there are ways you influence your home environment that are not as obvious. On a deeper and subtle level, our mental activity stimulates the atmosphere around us as well. Likewise, our cognitive processes have a range between still point and power point. Whether you are relaxed and enjoying the moment or recounting the frustrations from the day, your living space is influenced by your level of mental activity. Even though our thought processes can be very active, one reason that we do not notice this atmospheric influence is because we have also normalized to our own mental presence. We are accustomed to the range of internal conversations we have with ourselves every day, much like a fish in water.

One way to become more aware of the qualities projected by our own mental presence is to compare how we perceive our atmospheric environment in different situations. Now let us say that you are at home alone, and someone drops by for a visit. The moment this visitor enters your home, their presence alters the environment and you can perceive these changes. Obviously, you can see them, hear their voice, or any other sensations caused by their physical activity. However, have you ever noticed that there is something else that you detect? Your friend's arrival brings with it their mental activity that adds content to your atmospheric environment. Now there are *two* sources of mental activity, yours and theirs, emanating in the space around both of you. When this happens, the mental stimulations of the atmosphere entangle and share information.

Whether you are aware of this or not, most people acknowledge this entanglement in some way, even on a conscious level. Consider that almost immediately, you will make a judgment as to whether or not you find this person's presence enjoyable or unpleasant. You may even notice body sensations associated with your perception of their presence. These body sensations can range from feeling excitement or calm, feeling energetic or drained, based upon the level of ease or resistance you detect in their presence. Have you ever asked yourself *what* exactly is it that you are detecting?

There is more going on here than two thought fields bumping into each other as a result of proximity. Because what happens when someone else is present in your home but they are not in your proximity? Consider, for example, that they are sleeping in another room, and no interaction is occurring. In other words, there are no ordinary five physical sensory stimulations for you to detect to indicate their presence in your home. You know with your mind that they are there, but that knowledge is different from what you experience when you interact with them. Yet somehow, a perceptual difference lingers in the atmosphere. Your living space does not feel exactly the same to you as when you are home alone.

Here is another example. You arrive home from work after a long day. As you enter your home, are you able to determine whether or not someone else is there by the quality of the atmosphere you perceive? Is there someone sleeping or quietly relaxing in another room? In this situation, there is no five sensory information for you to detect. You cannot see them, hear them, smell them, taste them, or touch them, yet you still perceive their presence. So think about it. *What* exactly is it that you are detecting?

Some people might think I am referring to an aura, commonly thought of as a self-generated distinctive field that surrounds all people and objects. However, if the implication of an aura means it is self-generated, then it would travel with them wherever they go. Much the same way that a magnet carries its influence over metals wherever it goes rather than leaving its influence behind. If this is true, the moment the person leaves the room or the premises, then the perceptual shift that happens as a result of their physical presence should immediately cease. But if you think about this, you will realize that this is not what happens. Your environment continues to hold the changed atmospheric qualities that were perceived when the person was physically present. Over time, these qualities slowly fade and your home's atmosphere gradually returns to the ordinary state of stillness. Why does this happen, and what is the nature of these fading sensations?

One explanation is the longer our mental activity remains in a location, the stronger the atmospheric imprint. If we occupy a certain space with regularity, over time the atmosphere builds up memory from being continually stimulated by the same mental activity. For example, if you have siblings, children, or roommates living with you, pay a visit to their bedroom when they are not there. Have you noticed that you can perceive their presence even in their absence? Even after your sibling or children leave home for college or move out, the many years of their presence allows you to continue to feel their imprint in the atmosphere.

I propose that there is a layer of the atmosphere that responds to our thoughts. Even though I have used the words *mental activity* to describe the source that generates the thought atmosphere, our emotions contribute significantly to our thought content as well. Emotions tend to set our moods, and our moods often determine the thoughts we choose to have. As we emanate concentrations of thought in our proximity, this layer of the atmosphere responds by maintaining structure; remember, thought has sound and sound has form. People continually make deposits into a bank of data in the atmosphere that leaves behind a signature. This signature molds the atmosphere around us; much like clay is shaped with our hands. This layer of the atmosphere retains the shape of our thoughts even when we are no longer in vicinity. We move about in the world much like the weather and carry a force of influence over the atmosphere wherever we go. Usually, the influence dissipates soon after we leave a place where we spend little time. Much the same as when a storm passes through, we feel the residual effects of weather for a while, and then they slowly fade. However, in places that we frequent, such as our dwelling, the signature is deeply stamped by our consistent presence. Our influence over the atmosphere is significant for many reasons. In fact, many people will make real estate purchases based on these perceptions. Some people even report the ability to detect these atmospheric stimulations when they visit the home or bedroom of a loved one long after his or her death.

On one level, our influence is subtle, yet on another level, it is strong and substantial. We all have an innate awareness of these atmospheric stimulations because the language of thought, like the body indicators, is a language we all share. The degree to which we can interpret these atmospheric stimulations varies from person to person. Because of the subtle or delicate nature of these atmospheric stimulations, much depends on whether or not you have made developing your vocabulary a priority. You can choose to make it a priority at any time.

Beth's insistence to search my past for answers was starting to pay off. When I placed the lens of the indicators over the lens of the thought atmosphere, I peered through the body's kaleidoscope of health for the first time. The information I withheld when being tested in the study was making sense to me now. The vocabulary I had assembled, combined with detecting atmospheric qualities, had merged and matured and I was hearing what people's bodies were saying about the causes of their illness. I had discovered a very important piece to the puzzle. However, I was not sure how to put this information on a plate and serve it to Len and Beth. I decided to keep this information to myself a while longer.

Prominent Points for Chapter Review

- Every child begins with a boundless capacity for sensory perception.

- A standardized society insists on a collective experience that limits your sensory perception.

- Therefore, you are required to surrender some or all of your perceptual liberties in order to integrate into a standardized society.

- Shades of your perceptual past surface throughout your everyday life to remind you of your natural sensory capacities.

- Once you learn to recognize these perceptual prompts, you can begin to reclaim your natural sensory capacities.

Practical Application

Notice how you perceive the changes in your atmospheric environment as people enter and leave your home. Notice how long after their absence you continue to perceive their presence.

Compare your ability to detect changes in your atmospheric environment at home to other environments: place of work, library, restaurants, school, city streets, or your neighborhood.

Atmospheric stimulations are not limited to human beings. Other sentient creatures can cause stimulation. You can make perceptual observations about changes in the environment as a result of the presence of your house pets.

CHAPTER SIX

By the Numbers

I KEPT MY adventures in perception and health private from my family and most of my friends. However, professional development took me away from home more frequently; either I was in the Bethesda medical office working on the study, meeting with clients, or leading six-day residential seminars about perceptual expansion. The time away made it increasingly difficult to explain my nonattendance to my parents and friends. It took me several weeks to return phone calls, and that raised a lot of questions within my personal relationships. Excuses such as "I was mowing the lawn when you called" were no longer plausible.

Since my parents both came from traditional perspectives, I never told them about the night at the party when I was eight years old and the unfolding events thereafter. I was not sure if their conservative paradigms would accept this kind of information. But the time had come to pick up the phone and discuss the "real story" of the last three decades.

Surprisingly, my parents were inspired because they felt that assisting people with their health, no matter the method, was admirable. However, the conversation with my mother went on to reveal more clues to my mysterious medical mosaic.

Since she was curious about what I had said, I elaborated. When I told her how I see organ/system indicators of the body, she replied, "I know what you mean. I know what sarcoma of the uterus looks like." For once, it was my turn to be silent on the other end of the receiver. My mother was showing a side of herself she had not shared with me before. I asked her to explain to me what she saw. She said that she just knew "the look of sarcoma" as she called it, but she could not offer any details beyond her general description. She lacked a vocabulary to explain her perceptions. I could relate to her loss of words. My mother had learned to *see* sarcoma of the uterus because her mother had the illness during my mother's teenage years. My mother was the primary caregiver for her mother, and since they were together every day, she was constantly in the presence of the genital/

urinary indicator. She said that she could not see other illnesses as I could, but she knew the look of the loss of moisture and sarcoma. By the end of our conversation, receiving health information by looking at someone was not such a strange idea to her. As I hung up the phone, my mind whirled. I always *knew* I was not alone, but my mother confirmed what I had thought all along—people *can* see the indicators.

I had few friends in whom I confided my past and the clinical research. I had met Cliff a few years ago and although we did not get together very often, we kept in touch because of our shared interests in perceptual expansions. I told him about the medical study over the telephone. He was interested to hear more about our research and he suggested we get together for lunch. We met at a restaurant and I began to tell him about the unnoticed world of indicators.

Cliff asked me how I see the indicators when a couple sat down at a table nearby for lunch. My attention was quickly drawn to the woman and her neurological indicator, specifically pointing toward a stroke. The orchestration of events was perfect. I turned to Cliff and asked him to look at the woman and tell me what he saw. At first, he was not sure what I was asking him to do. He went through the standard description of hair color, clothing, posture, and so on. Then I asked him how it felt to be in her presence and could he make any other observations about her. After a few moments of observation, Cliff made the comment that she seemed to be a serious person and that she does quite a bit of intense *thinking*. I asked him to bring his attention to her forehead and if he could feel the *intense* thinking that radiated from her forehead much the same as heat radiates off the road in the horizon. Without hesitation, he responded, "Yes."

Next, I asked him to simply continue his observation and notice the connection between *looking* at the woman while *feeling* her thinking; how her thoughts permeated the atmosphere around her. I also told him to keep it simple, do not make the sensory experience more than what it is—simply relax and observe the *soft* activities and intricacies of the woman's *thinking* while maintaining his *visual* focus on her forehead. After a few moments of silent observation, Cliff nodded and then turned back to me and said that he remembered having the same sensation whenever he looked at his aunt just before she had her stroke.

With only a few minutes of guidance, it was easy for Cliff to identify the neurological indicator during a meal in a public restaurant. He even used some of the same adjectives I use to describe the neurological indicator. The confirmation I had been seeking was moving within reach, I had found another person who could see an indicator! I could not wait to share the news with Beth.

The next time I arrived to meet with Beth at the office, she was talking to a gentleman in the waiting room that I had never seen before; he was not a patient. It was not unusual for other health care providers to pay visits to Len and Beth for professional reasons. When Beth told them about our research study and what we were up to, of course, they wanted a demonstration of the assessment technique . . . on themselves. Beth and I obliged any opportunity to test the indicators for proficiency, and demonstrating the ease of applicability to members of the health care community was an added plus. Health care providers are people too, and I was surprised to discover how many of them experienced their own health imbalances with varying degrees of uncertainty or confusion. Perhaps their desire to solve their health problems prompted their career in health care. They were startled by how much I could tell them about their health without any knowledge of medical science or their health histories. The need for developing a methodical application of the indicators in the health care delivery system was becoming abundantly clear.

Although we kept this performance data separate from the clinical trials, we were gathering information from two sources—inside *and* outside the clinical study. These episodes were informal, but they were significant in two ways. First, I was presented with health imbalances I had not encountered in the study with immediate confirming feedback about the accuracy of the indicator. Second, the requests for spontaneous health assessments in a casual social setting demonstrated the ease of using the technique and allowed me to practice in front of a small audience. I did not know it at the time, but I was in another stage of preparation for what was to come: public demonstrations.

Once Beth's colleague left, I started to tell her about my discoveries with my mother and Cliff. But I was distracted by a woman who came into the office and sat down in the waiting room. Her body began sending me information about her health. As Beth and I made our way back to one of the examination rooms, I asked her, "Is that woman here to participate in the clinical study?"

"No, she is here for a regular medical appointment."

"She has a digestive indicator, but her moisture level is pretty high, so it most likely is not a serious digestive condition."

"John, can you explain to me exactly how you can see her condition? I know you talk about the different indicators, but that doesn't help me understand the process concretely. I want to know specifics."

"Okay, if you insist. It's the Helen Keller effect."

"What do you mean?"

"If you recall, at the age of nineteen months, Helen Keller lost her ability to see and hear. Her other senses of touch, smell, and taste came forward, and she learned to rely on only those three to navigate in the world. These three senses were much more sensitive to stimuli because of her loss of sight and hearing. When one of the five sensory inputs is compromised, the other senses can intensify their performance to make up for the deficit. For example, if you lost your ability to see, then your sense of hearing might become much more sensitive. The increased sensitivity to sound allows a person without the ability to see to notice sounds in ways that you and I do not. In this case, their 'noticing' magnifies their awareness of any audible sensations. People without the ability to see can pinpoint the proximity of objects in their environment, such as street traffic, people, doors and windows, and so on, without the sense of sight but with the sense of sound. They have learned how to hear *everything*."

"That might be true, but you have the full use of *all* your five senses. How does this compare?"

"Helen Keller's experience was initially a function of survival. At first, she had to learn how to make the same sensory distinctions about her environment with less than five senses in order to interact with the world. Her total sensory system adapted a level of performance almost identical to our five sensory capacities with only touch, taste, and smell. She learned to gather enough sensory data to navigate successfully in her environment. Once she satisfied her basic necessities for her survival, then she developed a vocabulary of sensory expression that was unique to her. However, she went on to develop recreational uses of her senses that allowed for social interaction and fun. She could communicate her experience to others about enjoying the beautiful day without seeing the sun, sky, trees, or meadow, or hearing the birds sing. Her sensory vocabulary allowed others to relate to her. Not only is Helen an example of sensory adaption, but she also shaped a world of perceptual reality that was uniquely hers and then made it available to others."

"Yes, I understand your point about sensory functions. I see where you are going with this, but that still doesn't tell me how to see health imbalances?"

"When we are very young children, we are infatuated by the world around us. Our curiosity wants to investigate every thing we encounter. Our primary sensory contact is usually a visual one. First, we see an object, and then we move in to investigate. Next, comes sensory follow-up, and that means we want to hold it, taste it, smell it. It's an inherent approach to constructing a world that we can understand. But mom and dad regulate our investigations by placing us in a play pen or crib. This is usually for safety reasons, so they give us approved items to examine called toys. But sooner or later, we're up for an entire household safari, and eventually, we escape the play pen to find a much bigger world of objects to investigate. But again, our period of investigation gets interrupted because it is not okay to touch and taste *everything*. Mom and dad still want to keep us safe, and that means control. This is where words such as 'children are to be seen, and not heard' and 'whatever you do, *don't* touch anything' get their life. So unless we disobey, all we are left with is the visual connection to the objects we admire in our proximity. Even though I examined items from a distance, my other senses came in for back up as an adjunct to vision in order to gather more sensory data. This is why I am sure that people have some experience of using their eyesight combined with other senses because we've all had to do it at some time in our lives. We've all had some version of not being able to touch the heck out of something we wanted to when we were very young. Since we couldn't touch it, we innately cast our other senses in front of us to make up for the loss of connection. We have already learned to feel at a distance through a visual channel, at least on an introductory level."

"So you are saying that you experienced some kind of selective sensory deprivation."

"Hmmm, since we are having this conversation, it would make sense that people who do not have the ability to see can make distinctions about the people they meet every day that you and I don't. They have learned to detect sensory data from other people without looking, but simply by standing in someone's presence, or from listening to the sound of someone's voice."

"Okay, so what happened next?"

"Along with our youthful infatuation comes incredible honesty. When I was a young boy, I believed that adults always meant what they said and said what they meant. After a series of disappointments because I had relied solely on the words of adults, it occurred to me that there is more to communication than what's being said. Listening solely to people's words was not providing me with enough information to determine the true intentions of their communication. My assessment was that I experienced a form of sensory deficit, and I needed to do something about it. I needed to cast my senses out in front of me and began fishing for more sensory data.

"There are many ways to perceive a person's communication, spoken or unspoken. I moved my attention away from listening to people's words and focused on body language and postures associated with different communication styles, but the ordinary use of my other senses really didn't provide me with any new information. This prompted me to go beyond the textbook use of my senses. I needed to adapt. I wondered if using my sense of hearing to listen in another way would be useful, and so I began the reinvention of my senses and how to use them from a multisensory state."

"What do you mean by a multisensory state? How did that show up in your perceptual world?"

"After examining my senses one by one, I arrived at a simple conclusion. My senses of smell and taste did not bring about any new areas of sensory applications. The act of sniffing or licking people may be a heaping spoonful to the senses of a dog, but it did not provide me with information beyond personal hygiene or detergent brand loyalty. So there were two senses left to combine with my sense of hearing: seeing and feeling. As children, the visual lens of our communication experience is primarily looking into the faces of people during conversations. That is where I began to focus my three remaining sensory receptors: seeing, feeling, and hearing.

"About the same time, I was learning about mathematics in grade school. My parents hired a tutor to give me lessons, and that included working with mathematical flash cards. I was learning the basics of addition and subtraction with the numbers one through ten. The tutor would hold the cards up with the equations written on the front so I could visually see the equations. It was during these lessons that I noticed a general 'visual feeling' when I looked at the cards. As time passed, I learned to distinguish that each number between one and ten had their own unique visual feeling. As the tutor pulled the cards, I associated the 'feeling' of the number with the correct answer to the equation. For example, if the flash card displayed $5 + 3$, I learned what an 8 felt like. It wasn't long before I could feel the answer when I looked at the card on top of the deck but *before* my eyes visually saw the equation."

"So you learned to translate data collectively among your different senses. The number eight looks like 8 or $5 + 3$ when using your eyes, but it also feels like . . . whatever it is you perceive with your feeling sense. An eight is the same either way. You are just using the different hardware to perceive it."

"Correct. However, although it sounds solely like a feeling sense, the use of my eyes was also essential. I played with the flash cards until I established a feeling vocabulary for each number. I reached a point where I could look at the printed patterns on the back of the cards, not the equations, and I was able to correctly identify the answers by the feel. But I needed to look at the card in order to do so. If I closed my eyes, it took much longer to feel the connection, and my accuracy was not as good. That's when I noticed my senses were blending, and that they needed to work together. What also made this easy was that I was only working with the numbers zero through ten. It was easy to derive ten distinct feelings. But as my skill level in mathematics advanced, and the answers to equations expanded to a range between zero and one thousand, there were too many feelings. The felt qualities about each number were too slight to distinguish, and to memorize them all would have been extremely difficult. Flash cards and numbers are inanimate while people are alive and full of characteristics. There is nothing wrong with learning from flash cards. But I stopped using them because I wanted to learn about people, not numbers. But I took what I learned from cards and returned my focus to identifying the intentions of people. After I learned to blend my senses, when I looked into the faces of people, I noticed that they projected sensations, much like the way you look at the sun and feel its radiation at the same time. But instead of radiant heat, I felt radiant characteristic, like the flash cards. Over time, I learned to make distinctions about these characteristics. That night at my parent's party when I saw the man with lung cancer, that's when it occurred to me that I was seeing the basic properties of health. Here I was looking for the truth within people's communication and found that what they truly communicate is their health. Ha! What a bonus!"

"Okay, so at this point, you are tuning in more clearly to your serendipitous discovery that people emit certain perceivable qualities that provide vital clues to their emotional and physical health. How did you learn to categorize and discriminate between the qualities?"

"There is a finite set of body organs and systems. If there were more than a hundred body organs, it would be more difficult to differentiate the characteristics, like the cards. Since there are roughly twenty major organs and systems, there are also approximately twenty different body indicators that I am aware of right now.

"During the study, I have made remarks that a health imbalance *was* more active in the past or *will be* more active in the future. The way I determine indicator activity and a time line is similar to feeling numbers on flash cards. Except now when I look at someone, any feelings of numbers signify months or years to me. If the number feels negative, it tells me the health activity is in the past. If the number feels positive, it's in the present or forward from this moment. There's more to it than that, but that's the best general way I can describe it to you."

"What about the woman in the waiting room? How did you know she has a digestive condition?"

"So, it's true. She does have a problem with her digestion."

"She is not participating in the study, so I am not going to discuss her health with you. But I still want you to explain to me. How have you detected that?"

"It's pretty obvious. I could see the indicators as soon as I walked in. Perhaps you see it, but you just don't know that you are."

"I see a woman sitting in a waiting room."

"Aha, that is because you are looking for something that isn't there. Since your eyes only show you a woman seated in a chair, you conclude there is nothing more to see. You haven't added the layers of the other senses. Don't look for more visual perception like clouds of colors or some kind of aurora borealis of the anatomy. Receive the ordinary image of the woman with your eyes, but don't *just look*. You must also *feel* with your eyes."

"How would you explain feeling with your eyes? How would I direct my experience to do that?"

"Look across the room at the door and tell me if it is made of a soft or hard material."

"It is a hard material—it's made of wood."

"But how is that you can report a 'hard' assessment of the door without touching it?"

"I can see that it is made of wood, and I know that wood is a hard material from touching it. But this is a function of my experience of my ordinary senses and from memory."

"Ah, you're expecting this to come to you through some new kind of vision, a new kind of sense. I keep telling you that it will come to you through the ways that you already use your senses. There is nothing special here. Don't discount your memory of what objects feel like to you either.

Once you learn the indicators, you will need to store the sensory experience in your memory that will allow you to recognize the indicators whenever you encounter them again, just like your memory of the hard door."

"I can understand the concept, but I am still not sure I understand it as you intend me to."

"This is simple, but I did not say this would be easy. But perhaps direct experience would work better for you. Let's play with this. The digestive indicator is pretty easy indicator for me to identify, so perhaps it will be easy for you, too. That might be a good place for you to start."

"What do you mean?"

It was at this point that I finally had the chance to tell her about the conversations with my mother and Cliff.

After I told her, she said, "Well, can you teach me in a way that I can understand it?"

"Let's find out. If the patient in the study today has a digestive indicator after I finish my assessment and we satisfy the testing protocol, I want you to sit with the patient and me for a few minutes. Just notice as much as you can about the patient, and we'll see if your description reveals the digestive indicator."

Fortunately, the patient to be examined that day in the clinical study did have a digestive indicator. She had a few other indicators as well, but I felt that the digestive indicator was prominent enough to put Beth's perceptions to the test. Since the other indicators were mild, it would be easy to draw her attention to what I wanted her to see. After the patient left, Beth and I resumed our conversation.

"Okay, so what did you notice about her?"

"Well, I am not exactly sure what you mean. Her complexion was clear but somewhat dim. Her eyes looked tired, she did not seem to have much energy or enthusiasm. She sat in the chair with poor posture. Is that what you mean?"

"Let's take another approach. Rather than you guessing, I am going to lead you quickly down a path. Tell me more about the dimness in her complexion."

"Well . . . there was a dimness . . . a darkness . . ."

"Please continue."

"What else is there to say about it? She had darkness. It seemed like her complexion had a shadow on it."

"Are you saying the room was dimly lit, or the fluorescent light cast a shadow on her face? We are sitting in the exact same light as when you looked at her. Do I have the same shadow on my complexion?"

"No, you don't."

"Rather than say that her complexion had a shadow on it, would a more accurate description be that the shadow seemed to *generate* from her complexion?"

"Well . . . yes . . . now that you mention it, I could describe it in those terms."

"And you detected this shadow by looking at her face?"

"Yes."

"Would you say that it projected, that the shadow 'radiated' from her complexion?"

"Yes, the word *radiate* would describe how I perceive this shadow . . . this darkness."

"That's confirming. Many of the indicators have what I would call radiant qualities."

"Okay, but what's your point?"

"I am not a scientist, but I can make some generally accepted scientific statements about what I think is going on. All things are made of matter, which is composed of atoms made up of electrons, protons, and neutrons. These atoms are in a perpetual state of vibration with varying rates that arrange the different states of matter—gases, liquids, and solids. The molecules vibrate on a microscopic scale and at such a fast rate that our eyes do not detect their motion. Our experience of matter is one of the three states, but the molecules are vibrating all the time nonetheless."

"Okay, so where are you going with this, John?"

"One result of this vibration is that all matter has a certain level of radiation. I do not mean dangerous levels of radioactivity, but that all matter releases vibratory emanations on a microscale. You must learn to feel this radiation, much the same as feeling the warmth radiated by the sun on your face. Or the way you can feel the vibration of a beating drum. Is her complexion the only place on her body that the darkness radiates from?"

"I don't know. Was I supposed to pay attention to somewhere else?"

"Let's take another approach. I know this may not be easy since you are working from memory. If she was seated in the room right now, it would probably be easier. But if you are going to apply this skill effectively, you will need to know how to work from memory. Because once you remember how the indicators feel, you can recall the information any time, much like remembering how a wooden door feels. Can you remember what it was like when she was sitting here, the feel of her presence? Keep in mind that her digestive indicator is not a severe one. It is not a third degree. Give yourself some sensory latitude. I have already asked you to explore your senses. Perhaps what you need to explore first is the permission to explore the senses. Conceptualize what it would feel like if you could put your hand through the door and feel the grain of the wood from the inside. Then apply that same concept to what the radiation of this darkness would feel like."

"Okay, I can do that. I am also starting to understand what you mean by blending your senses. First, using my eyes to perceive by seeing and then exploring that already-formed image with a deeper sense of feeling. This sort of feeling has a tactile quality to it, but I am not using the touch receptors in my hands to perceive it."

"How would you describe the dimness, the darkness, to me? Would you say that it is a surface darkness, or does it seem to be sourced deeper, that it actually radiates from beneath her complexion?"

"Yes, it feels to me like it radiated from beneath her complexion."

"Okay, now follow the emanation to the source, and tell me where it takes you?"

"Now that you mention it, it includes both her complexion and her torso, but not her extremities. In fact, it is sourced in her torso and emanates through the entire region from her abdomen to her face. It is mostly concentrated in the abdomen, but it is the face that provides me with the sensation of the emanation. Logically, my eyes are drawn to her abdomen to get information about her digestion. But looking at her abdomen does not give me the same sensation as when I look at her face. It's like looking into a tuba. I must connect with the emanation from her face in order to perceive the sensation from her abdomen."

"Precisely, now let's return to the darkness itself. Tell me more about the darkness."

"Well, it's just dark. That's all, but you are not going to let me get away with that vague of a description, are you?"

"Look again, there are different kinds of darkness, and you are learning how to see many different kinds of qualities; different intensities of darkness."

"Okay, I can understand that, but can you give me some more guidance?"

"Believe it or not, I am asking you to feel what a digestive system in discord feels like. You have located the source. Now you must examine the content. Does it have a dense, thick quality to it, or does it have a sparse or light porous quality?"

"It has a dense thickness to it."

"Exactly!"

"That's it? That's an indicator?"

"Yes, see, I told you it's not supernatural. And the more intense and dense the dark thick feeling is, the more severe the condition. If I tell you that you have just perceived a mild dark thickness, does that make sense to you?"

"Yes, it does."

"Now that you know how it feels, does it also give you a sense of how a person's compromised digestion feels? Can you associate the dark thickness with the biological environment of the body's compromised digestive tissues?"

"Yes, I can."

"Think about how other illnesses such as colon cancer, diverticulosis, or IBS might feel in the body. Can you sense a mild darkness for IBS and a severe darkness for an invasive tumor?"

"Hmmm . . . right now, I don't have enough experience with this process to know for sure that I can perceive cancer, but I am with you so far with *mild*."

"Congratulations, Beth, you have just learned your first indicator."

"Believe it or not, now that you brought this to my attention, this is something I have noticed working with some of my patients over the years . . . but I didn't know that it meant anything. That wasn't too difficult. Can you teach me another indicator?"

"They may not all be this easy at first. I did not learn the entire set of indicators in a week. I selected the digestive indicator to start with because from my perspective it is one of the easier ones to learn. There are some that are more challenging. Let's practice with your ability to blend your senses together successfully and work with some of the other simple indicators for now. Later, we can get to the ones that are more complex to identify."

"Okay, so how do I practice?

"Beth, it's time you and I take a field trip."

Prominent Points for Chapter Review

- Everyone has the ability to perceive health indicators.

- While we have commonly shared perceptual styles in a standardized society, we also have unique perceptual styles that developed during childhood based on individual environment, circumstances, needs, and interests that lie dormant.

- By using the standards of society as a basis for sensory experience, we can reintroduce unique perceptual styles into the standardized sensory base of knowledge, thus, creating hybrid sensory techniques.

- The process of perceiving health indicators is a teachable/learnable skill.

Practical Application

- Obtain a deck of mathematical flash cards.

- You may perform this exercise alone or with a partner.

- Begin with equations that have an answer between one and ten.

- Shuffle the cards and place them on the table in front of you, or have someone hold the card in front of you. (The reason I don't want you to hold the card is so you do not let the feeling sensation you are seeking have anything to do with the weight of the card. You must learn to feel without physical contact.)

- Calculate the correct answers to the equation.

- Looking at the equation and knowing the answer, experiment with the combination of your sense of sight and touch. For example, if the flash card before you shows 5+3, set the intention of knowing how the number 8 feels. You may have a felt sensation in your body, or you may notice a felt quality about the atmosphere around you.

- Continue with this practice until you have a sense of how the numbers one thru ten feel to you from a combined sensory perspective.

- Once you are comfortable with the sensations associated with the different numbers, place the deck in front of you without looking at the equations. Based upon your memory of the feeling of the numbers, determine the answer *before* you look at the equation on the card.

This application is intended to create a feeling sensation with the eyes. Attempting to see the number through the cards or in your mind's eye is an entirely different practice.

CHAPTER SEVEN

Riding the Bike

WE NEEDED TO expose Beth to as many indicators as possible in the shortest amount of time. Observing one or two people per day as I did during the clinical trials was not going to put Beth on the fast track to unfolding her own sensory potential. The location needed to be a place where we could observe a large number of people up close without interruption. Weather could not be a factor; an indoor site would be required. Beth and I looked at each other, and the answer quickly became obvious to us—the shopping mall.

We set a day and a time to meet and began Beth's education of the indicators. Initially, we walked around from store to store looking at people while they shopped. The mall was an ideal classroom for creating awareness about the health indicators because there were many people who projected a wide variety of health imbalances. At first, I pointed out those who demonstrated intense or third-degree indicators to make it easy for her to see, or so I thought. But the many different qualities demonstrated by the people at the shopping mall sent her whirling.

"Look, Beth, there's a cardiovascular indicator in Men's Shoes. Over in Cosmetics, there is a liver indicator. Quickly, Beth, the woman in the red hat near the restaurant. She has an infertility indicator and a blood glucose indicator."

Beth spun in circles to keep up with my directives as though she was in some kind of perceptual pinball game. The mixture of different health indicators was too much. Since this was the beginning of her teaching, pointing at the indicators as they rapidly passed by failed to provide the foundation piece I was seeking. People did not stand still long enough for Beth to learn how to identify much of anything.

After a few hours of wandering through the mall without success, we decided to make it easier on our feet and positioned ourselves on a bench at the bottom of an escalator. Our new station gave Beth's eyes more time to observe each person and experiment with adjusting her senses. While everyone has a prior experience base with their senses, not everyone is on the exact same page; people absorb their experiences at variable rates. To develop an expert command of the indicators during an afternoon trip to the mall would be equivalent to completing a doctorate in medicine in a single day. Without being certain of what she was actually looking for and bounding from one health indicator to another, she was inundated with sensory data she could not sort. We needed a common point of origin and reference. We took a break for lunch to discuss our next step.

"Let's get back to basics, Beth."

"Okay."

"Communication is all around us, and it can take a variety of forms, but most importantly, communication is a skill. For example, what we call body language is a nonverbally expressed language that people speak whether they are aware of it or not. We didn't go to body language school when we were kids, yet it is a form of communication that has emerged in most every culture. But here is where the interpretation of communication can split because not everyone agrees upon what the body language means. People can have different interpretations that they derive from the body actions of others. For instance, if a person has their arms folded across their chest in a closed-body position, for some people, this could mean that the person is personally unavailable, not approachable. Or it could simply mean the room temperature is cold, and they are responding to their environment with their body posture. It may have nothing to do with their approachability. My point is that two people can observe the same body language, and yet arrive at two vastly different interpretations. The success to developing an accurate skill of body language is by aligning your interpretations with the intention behind the sent message.

"The body indicators are also a form of communication that has emerged in all cultures. But it has all gone unnoticed because of the wide variance in people's interpretations, plus people have never been told that the indicators were there to begin with. I see the exact same optical image as you when we both look at people. The only difference is that you see people walking by, and I see health imbalances walking by."

"I am not so sure about that."

"Unless I can create useable imagery or ideas that are familiar to you through your ordinary five senses, we won't get very far. You must learn to connect the ordinary use of your perception with the ordinary events of the day and make extraordinary distinctions. Are you really getting the most out of every perceptual experience? It is in the overlooked places where you will find raw stimuli that are translatable through your ordinary senses. Until now, you just haven't paid close attention to it. This isn't sixth sensory stuff, I am simply asking you to place your awareness on your unawareness.

"Let's break this down even further, Beth. Communication probably began as hand signs or gesture, verbal noises, then the spoken word, and eventually, the written word. Primarily, people communicated in the presence of one another. To make a very long history short, technologies developed to the point that communication could travel through wire by means of the telegraph. It was no longer necessary to conduct communication in proximity to one another. Next, the advent of radio and television brought communication to a wireless state. Sound and picture were converted into a signal that could travel on the airwaves unseen by anyone in its path. No one has ever reported seeing television waves traveling through their living room into their television set. Now, in our time, the airwaves are saturated with communication traffic. E-mail, Internet data, and cellular communications have increased the amount of information that travels in the bandwidth of our planetary atmosphere. Huge amounts of data and programming language are fluttering around us at this very moment right here in this mall. Even though it is completely unobserved by anyone, it is present and active nonetheless. Our computer age has actually brought forward the vocabulary we have lacked over the centuries to describe the capabilities of the senses. In other words, electronic telepathy, data in its crudest binary form, ones and zeros, are freely traveling back and forth. It requires a receptor, or a computer, to receive this disarray of data and reassemble its binary code into characters of text that form words and convey meaning.

"My point is that communication itself hasn't really changed all that much. It is only the channels or methods by which information travels that have matured and become more complex. People accept without difficulty that information can travel through the atmosphere from one handheld device to another. But as soon as you suggest that information can travel from one human being to another, people are up in arms shouting 'Horse hockey!' Currently, you receive medical communication in the form of blood tests, X-rays, and so on. Now, you are simply widening your bandwidth to receive the same medical information through another channel, one that is instantly available."

"But if I don't detect this information, how I am going to receive it?"

"Just as electronic data can ride the atmosphere, so can your perceptions. We are specifically working with biological data, and since your body is biological, you are already designed to transmit and receive information through your own biology. The program is already on your hard drive, so to speak. Now you must install it. Your body already knows how to speak this language. It is time to connect this ability to your awareness."

"But there must be something new and different about all this."

"Perhaps, but I'll bet you have never sat down with yourself and decided that you were going start using your senses differently, in a new way, even if it is only ever so slightly. Most people aren't interested in a series of incremental phenomenon. They are waiting for something big, something really fantastic to happen. But seldom is an epiphany enough to alter one's perception indefinitely. The real transformation occurs *after* the epiphany. It is the day-to-day living with the commitment to maintain what the epiphany has illuminated—that's the real challenge. You need to allow your world of the senses to change, and therefore, the rules must also change, but that does not come about by simply 'changing your mind' because of some transcendental event. Nor does this depend upon repeating some daily affirmations, such as 'I can do this, I can do this.' Yes, it's important to affirm your desire to do so, but there has to be gold backing the currency. You can jump up and down all you want and declare that you are going to ride the bicycle, but when you first get on you will probably fall down several times. We begin one pedal stroke at a time and move toward balance, along with determination to replace the internal conversations about the reality in which you live. Your words must come into alignment with your actions, your experiences, which is not the same as changing your mind or reciting an affirmation script. The internal conversation I have with myself says I can see health imbalances, and somewhere in your internal conversation lives doubt or resistance because you want these perceptions to come on your terms, on your rules of reality. But that reality does not grant permission. The only difference between you and me right now are these two conversations. Everything else, including seeing the indicators, is just a detail that becomes available when you release how you have been conditioned to understand certain kinds of experiences. Before we go any further, the question you need to ask yourself is do you *really* want your reality to change? You won't learn to see indicators while keeping all your old rules about reality and the way life *is* intact. That's why I say this is simple but not easy. Because most people believe that their reality, their world view, is the right one. Most people aren't in any hurry to let go of the beliefs they hold so dearly. But there isn't much room for anything else to happen if their cup is already full.

"We need to bring your experiences into alignment with your true desire to access indicators. Your interest to know all this is linked to a much larger desire you have—to nurture people by providing them with the best health information possible so, ultimately, they can heal. But you may be in conflict because you want the best of both worlds. You want to see indicators so you can provide people with the best health care possible, but you don't want any *other* rules of your reality to change. You are at a choice point because once you open this door, there is no going back, only forward. Once you learn to perceive the indicators, you will see them from that moment on. Yes, you can ignore them but once stretched, your perception will never return to its previous dimension.

"Since this is day one for both of us, me teaching and you learning, let's simplify this as much as possible. Remember, you are not going to experience some kind of transcendental state. This comes through your five physical senses and through the imagery you create in your mind from the experience of your five physical senses. *Intuition* or *psychic* are just words people use when they cannot describe how they perceive something that they can't fully explain. However, I say it's just another way of using your senses. You've had a lifetime of people shining their indicators at you. Now it's time to feel the sun. These perceptual sensations can be mild or intense, but maybe the individual 'trees' of the indicators are so close to your face you cannot see them. Let's take a few steps back and begin to see through the forest of perception."

"Your philosophy behind all this makes perfect sense to me, but in general, I am really not sure just what it is that I am looking for. You keep saying this is a matter of noticing and communicating, but how am I supposed to notice and receive this communication?"

"Since you are not confident about what to look for or how to look just yet, let's go back to that day in your office when you were able to identify the digestive indicator. Since you already have some experience with the digestive indicator, you have an idea of what you're looking for. Let's set our sights on identifying only digestive imbalances today. Once you have a clear sense of how to see one of the indicators, then we can move on to expanding your indicator vocabulary."

Beth agreed.

We returned to our post at the base of the escalator, except this time, I only identified people with digestive indicators. This allowed extended time for Beth to remain in a perceptual mode with her focus on the dark thickness of the digestive indicator. We observed all degrees of digestive conditions over the next few hours. I pointed out severe or third-degree indicators to her initially, and we worked our way toward mild conditions. By the end of the day, she had a firm understanding of the full range of first-degree to third-degree digestive indicators with proficiency. She also learned the distinction between an upper and lower intestinal tract indicators; upper intestinal conditions are evidenced by a light dark thickness, and lower intestinal conditions are heavy dark thickness. This process of teaching worked very well, and Beth was excited with her results.

The rate at which Beth grasped an understanding of the indicators was promising. A few weeks later, we returned to the mall to learn the next indicator—respiratory. Beth struggled at first because she thought she would see the respiratory indicator as easily as the digestive. When I asked her to describe how she perceived the respiratory indicator, I quickly realized she thought that she would feel the respiratory indicator in exactly the same way as the digestive indicator. The only difference she thought would be that it would be seen in another region of the body.

"I understand that I need to be open, but give me more technique, give me more 'how to,'" she said.

"Before I came to your office in November 2001, I had already considered how to teach this to people. Since your body can generate indicators, it can also receive indicators, but the vocabulary is broad, so don't try to feel each indicator exactly the same. Allow your senses to roam. Imagine a sliding scale with eyesight at one end of the spectrum and feeling at the opposite end. Some indicators are more visually based while others are more kinesthetically based. You must learn to move along this sensory scale from end to end as you desire. As you move, let your body become a receptor to the kind of stimuli this blended state allows, like a thermometer. But instead of detecting levels of heat, you are detecting textures. Next, multiply this receptivity. Instead of one thermometer, you become a series of thermometers, much like a harp with each string set to resonate with a certain pitch. Here's another point of reference. With the digestive indicator, the position on the sensory scale is approximately 70 percent visual, 30 percent feeling. You can see it and feel it at the same time. As you work with the respiratory indicator, move more into your sense of feeling so that you are about 65 percent visual and 35 percent feeling. I know this may sound like an insignificant difference, but these are the kinds of intricate distinctions you're going to have to make."

"Easier said than done."

"We talked about blending your senses and becoming a receptor. Connect these two ideas and engage them at the same time."

"Tell me more about how to feel with my eyes."

"Recall feeling the wooden door from a distance. This time, I want you to think of cooking at home in your kitchen. Bring to mind when you make a dry seasoning mix. Think of mixing a half cup of salt with a half cup of pepper in your hands. What does it feel like to hold this mixture in your hands, the sensations of a gritty substance as the fine grains fall through your fingers? Can you connect with this memory? Let me know when you're there."

"I'm there."

I waited until I observed someone descending the stairs with a respiratory indicator.

"Now *as you look* at that gentleman coming down the escalator while connecting or recalling this memory of feeling the texture of salt and pepper in your hand, can you see *and* feel that he has an ashy texture in his upper torso region and face. Use your eyes the same way that you look at a door across the room and know that it is hard without touching it. Careful now, the respiratory indicator is not dark and thick, like the digestive indicator. There is no density. This time, the indicator is arid and porous like the salt and pepper in your hands. *Look* and *feel* the salt and pepper."

"Yeeessssssss!" Beth suddenly exclaimed. "I can see it. I mean I feel it. I mean . . . I got it!"

After a few more field trips to the mall, Beth had learned to detect four indicators: digestive, respiratory, thyroid, and blood glucose. But what impressed me the most was how quickly she was able to identify the Life Span Moisture Level. Not only could she identify the severe loss of moisture, but she could assign moisture percentage values to anyone she looked at with nearly identical accuracy to mine. As a health care provider, having the command of detecting the Life Span Moisture Level would be invaluable to her patients. Beth's perceptions became more attuned to recognizing these indicators, and she continued to fine-tune her skills in public. I no longer pointed out indicators to her as I did in the beginning. Eventually we reversed roles, and I waited for her to inform me of an indicator as we walked down the street together.

Beth was pleased with her progress, but there was one important element missing to her learning process—feedback. We never approached any of the people we observed in public to find out if they had a condition that related to the indicators she observed. Although I was convinced of her abilities, protocol dictated feedback, and without it, the successes at the mall were all conjecture. It was time for her to return to her medical practice, make these observations for herself, and receive feedback via her patients and clinical medical tests.

And that is exactly what she did. It was not long before I received phone calls at home from Beth about observing the indicators of her patients in the waiting room, noting the indicator intensities, and then confirming her observations when she met with the patients in the examination room minutes later.

Sometimes though when we spoke, Beth was frustrated because she encountered health imbalances in patients that she had not yet coupled to an indicator. Without knowing how to identify the imbalance she perceived, all she could see was the forest. She knew the body was showing her a tree, but she did not know what it meant.

On one occasion, she called to tell me what happened while flipping through the pages of a popular magazine. A story had caught her attention about a well-known television cooking show host. The article was about the chef's latest announcement of suddenly changing his style of cuisine. He now advocated diabetic delicacies and how to prepare full flavorful meals for those who have diabetes. Beth concluded the chef's motivation for the modification of cuisine must be due to the fact that he had developed adult onset diabetes, which altered his style of cooking. But when Beth looked at the recent photographs of the chef in the magazine, she was not able to detect the diabetes indicator. Up until this point, Beth was confident with her ability to identify the diabetic indicator and had received successful feedback in her office on several occasions. She was stymied by the photograph and questioned her ability to detect the indicator. She told me that she reviewed the photograph of the chef over and over, and no matter how many times she adjusted her senses when looking at the snapshot, she kept coming up with nothing.

Disappointed with her inaccurate assessment, she finished reading the article anyway. But when she turned the last page of the article, there on the next folio was a photograph of a woman that Beth clearly recognized as projecting the diabetes indicator. She read the final text of the article, and the woman in the photograph was the wife of the television chef. The article explained that as a result of his wife having diabetes, he had changed his cuisine to support her dietary needs. Subsequently, he wanted to educate people about how a diabetic diet does not mean boring, bland food. People can have a diabetic diet with a variety of spices and flavors.

Since these visual assessments are nonintrusive and only require looking at someone, Beth and I could engage our indicator awareness in any social situation. Although these episodes were not included in the formal study, they were invaluable nonetheless. Whenever we met with friends or colleagues, we received more feedback about the indicators simply by asking them about their health. Once again, new information was revealed when we encountered health imbalances that were not in any of the patients in the clinical trials.

"Beth, the gentleman on the other side of the room has a cardiovascular indicator, but there is something unusual about the way it is projected."

"Do you mean there is something different about his indicator that is not consistent with those whom you have perceived the cardiovascular indicator?"

"No, the indicator is the same, but the way that it is projected is altered. It shakes or vibrates. It's there, but it's as though it won't take hold. I have seen indicators behave like this in the past, but I haven't been able to find out what it means."

"I know this gentleman, John. Let's ask him, and maybe he can tell us something that will help us to understand more deeply."

Beth talked with the man, and he said that cardiovascular diseases had been present in his ancestral lineage. Although his father had a history, to his knowledge, he was free of any cardiovascular disease.

"John, do you suppose this shake or vibration in the indicators could point to hereditary health conditions?"

"Well, I have seen this before with people I know, and that might explain why I have noticed indicators that don't seem to fully take hold, and the person never develops an illness."

"When the indicators vibrates or won't take hold, as you described, it means that the health condition runs in the family, but the person does not necessarily have the condition?"

"It's possible, but I haven't been tested for detecting hereditary health imbalances in the study, so I can't say for sure."

"If it's true, this information would be useful. If a certain disease runs in a family then members want to know if they will contract the disease as well. But this reaches beyond just heredity. Could it be that the body has a way of knowing if it will *ever* contract a disease? Does the body's awareness extend that far into the future?"

"Yes, and remember, there are modifiers that do not relate to a certain body organ or system but tell me about the overall health imbalance. They augment the indicator information."

"What else can these modifiers tell you?"

"There is one modifier that I call an extreme modifier. It does not mean that a person has an extreme health imbalance, but I have given it this name because of how I perceive it. It looks extreme. Whenever I see this modifier, I know that the health imbalance is uncommon and that it will not be a straightforward diagnosis for a physician. Medical science can not take an ordinary approach to this kind of situation, or it will likely miss the correct diagnosis. For example, if I see someone with a muscular/skeletal indicator, a loss of moisture, *and* an extreme modifier, it is probably a rare form of bone or tissue cancer. Normal cancer tests may not detect the illness. Once again, the delay of proper treatment can make all the difference in these instances. The sooner they know, the sooner they can proceed with effective treatments. The same treatment may not be effective at a later date, and most physicians would agree that time is a critical factor when it comes to cancer treatment."

"What does an extreme modifier look like?"

"I am not sure exactly how the extreme modifier could be illustrated on paper. I can only point it out to you when I see it. So far, as we have been working together, I have not seen the extreme modifier, but I will let you know when I do."

"Okay, are there more than two modifiers?"

"There is another modifier I call sudden-death. I can probably count on one hand the times I have seen it, but when I have, death has occurred within a few days, or death is swift and unexpected. It doesn't have anything to do with moisture levels. This modifier tells me that a sudden shock to the body system will occur. Or at least that is what I have been able to determine from what I have seen and the feedback I received about the news of their death. I can only speculate about the people I see on the street because I never receive any feedback. I am also not sure how I would illustrate a sudden-death modifier, I can only show you when I see it."

"Give me an example of the sudden-death modifier. What happened?"

"It was several years ago at my place of work. We had a new person join our work team in the office. I met him on Monday morning, and when I returned to work on Thursday, he had died from hepatitis. Other than the modifier, his appearance was normal. If you saw him, you probably would not have noticed anything. I know this may sound contradictory, but his moisture level was in the normal range and he died anyway."

"Hepatitis is a virus-related health imbalance. Not a body born illness or growth like cancer. Perhaps that is why it did not show up in the moisture level. Can you identify other viruses?"

"Our clinical study is the only testing I've had so far. I haven't been tested for viruses, but I have encountered them with some of the people I know. For example, the herpes virus still shows up to me as a genital/urinary indicator, at least I know it does in women. It doesn't tell me it's a virus, just that there is some kind of imbalance with the sex organs. I am not sure how it would show up in men."

"John, can you see AIDS?"

"Yes and no. I don't know much about medical science's research of AIDS, only what I have heard from newspapers and television, so my information may or may not comply with conventional wisdom. But I can tell you about AIDS from an indicator perspective. There may be more than one strand of AIDS virus. The reason I say that is because after looking at several people who told me they have the AIDS virus, I thought I had determined the indicator. Later, I met people who told me they had the virus, and I *did not* see the indicator. Then I saw someone with the indicator, and they *did* have the virus. Perhaps they were receiving treatment at the time and that reduced the indicator visibility. Or maybe I have learned the indicator for one kind of AIDS virus, but there could be other strands. What is interesting to me is that AIDS does not show up as a blood indicator. It closely resembles the infertility indicator in women. I am curious to know if infertility is related to an immune deficiency rather than a dysfunction of the reproductive organs. Or the opposite may apply. What can we take from what we know about infertility and apply that to AIDS research? Beth, what feedback can you give me about what you know about the behavior of viruses?"

"Medical science says . . ."

Beth continued to report to me about her feedback while meeting with her patients. There were also times when she called to say how *unhappy* she was that she was accurate. One gentleman who came to see her was literally losing moisture before her eyes. She called me a few weeks after seeing him to tell me he died. These moments of sorrow in the study were few, and we both knew that working in the health profession meant there would be news like this. Beth also knew how important it was to accurately observe the Life Span Moisture Levels if she wanted to perform a comprehensive health assessment with her patients. But Beth was not alone, the knowledge of indicators would soon bring sadness to my own life.

Over time, phone calls and e-mails arrived at my home with news of family and friends afflicted with health conditions. At first, the health problems were moderate in nature, and friends or extended family were receiving treatment. Then the day came when I received an e-mail about my friend Reese who demonstrated the aggressive loss of Life Span Moisture Level that pointed to cancer more than ten years ago. The e-mail described how she had been in the hospital for a month in a medically induced coma to stabilize her systems. She already had several surgeries, and much of her intestinal tract had been removed because of an invasive growth. I deeply regretted having not said anything, but how do you tell someone they will have cancer in ten years? Would anyone have believed me? For the first time in my life, I did not want to see illness when I looked at people. The heat of tears was building. I could not finish reading the words in the e-mail. I closed my eyes and wept.

Prominent Points for Chapter Review

- Negotiating your sensory perceptions is similar to learning how to ride a bicycle.

- The ability to ride a bicycle lives within each one of us.

- You must find *your* equilibrium in the face of many sensory variables.

- There will be times when you fall down.

- You find your equilibrium by falling down.

- There are times when you will believe you have fallen down when you have not.

CHAPTER EIGHT

Close to Home

ONCE REESE WAS home from the hospital, I went to visit her. I wanted to support my friend in any way that I could. The human spirit is prone to endurance even in the face of tremendous adversity. Although it's much more challenging in the later stages of illness, it is never too late to address the indicators and the thought atmosphere.

When she answered the door, my heart sank. She was losing moisture rapidly, and her whole body system was in chaos. Since there were several family members present I could not speak with her openly. We only had a few minutes to visit so I had to work quickly. I focused my attention on her indicators and thought atmosphere while we spoke. But she was severely traumatized from the combination of the illness, medical procedures and medications that her body was struggling for survival at the very core.

I waited for the opportunity to speak to her privately so I could share with her the information that her body was telling me. Unfortunately, she was highly medicated, and her attention wandered. She could not focus for more than a few seconds and switched topics quickly, at times in mid-sentence. I was not sure if she comprehended or remembered what we discussed. She spoke of younger days and the fun we had shared together. I waited for her thoughts to focus, but five minutes were all we had together. I left without being able to communicate to her what I could see. As I walked toward my truck, I knew her health and future were in her hands, not mine. The same way that Rhonda's symptoms hindered her from working on her personal power struggle, the amount of biological devastation Reese had experienced would make it very difficult to connect with the messages from her body. This visit was our last time together; she passed away shortly after.

Sadness continued as I received more news of friends and relatives diagnosed with terminal illness. In some cases, indicators I had observed during holiday gatherings when I was in my teens had finally come to pass. These instances provided more evidence of the body indicator's early warning capabilities, with more and more occurrences of indicators being present decades in advance of a diagnosis; I was uncertain of the most effective way to conduct my private sessions with people. Without any signs or symptoms evident, many people resisted the idea that illness was in their future even though the indicators were already present. My sole purpose for working with people was to convey their body's message and initiate their own recovery process before an illness could set in but that was not happening. I continued to search for the best way to get them proactively involved in their health.

§ § §

Beth had similar experiences with resistance in the conventional health care delivery system. After completing her masters of science in nursing, she worked in a conventional medical practice. She recognized there were other aspects to people's health and well-being that went beyond physiology. She noticed that many patients would not follow the health recovery recommendations set forth during office visits, whether it was not taking medications properly, not returning to the office for additional visits, not pursuing further treatments, or following up with a specialist for care. The list of ways that people abandoned their healing process was endless, and so were the reasons. Beth firmly believed as I did that many patients were not going to heal unless they reconciled the dysfunction of their interpersonal relationships with others or with self no matter how many drugs were prescribed. She also felt her Hippocratic Oath had not been honored by sending people packing with pills.

She was not alone in her conviction. Many of her health care colleagues were frustrated by this conservative approach, and they too wanted to engage the deepest aspects of healing. The limited interactive structure had been set forth by the conventional health care delivery system. Beth demanded more from medicine, and she wanted to break the chains that bound her patients to their self-defeating behaviors and, ultimately, their illness. She could no longer stand still and wear the conservative mask of medicine. After years of dissatisfaction, her quest for practicing a broader spectrum of health care led her to seek other medical approaches.

The desire to address the totality of people's health called her to practice what she was learning. When Beth completed Gestalt therapy training, her profession as a health care provider dramatically transformed. She left her conventional practice and joined Dr. Wisneski as an integrative nurse practitioner. She was now free to engage all aspects of being—physical, emotional, intellectual, and spiritual—when she worked with patients.

I often wondered how Beth could participate in our unconventional clinical study without raising a brow. She had taken my process and concepts in stride, and now I knew why. She had been exploring the psychospiritual aspects of health and disease long before I arrived at her Bethesda office. Beth and I finally came to realize how much we had shared a common goal all along—to provide people with the most valuable information available so they could propel their journey of healing forward.

But why would a person avoid information that could restore their health? What reasons would a person hold themselves hostage to their own illness? Perhaps people become comfortable with what they do not know or with what they *pretend* to not know. If illness has been incorporated into someone's thought atmosphere and people become invested or attached to the drama or reality it offers, the removal of even a small piece of that drama can be very threatening to their identity.

§ § §

Beth and I continued to search my past for answers. But it kept coming back to the simple fact that my childhood reeked of curiosity. With the cognitive development of a child as my only ally, the natural reach of the senses made perfect sense to me. On the other hand, without anyone to talk to, I remained curious, and that pulled me forward. As Beth prodded for more answers, eventually, our conversations came around to some of the other experiences that youth had to offer besides indicators.

I stated earlier that there were no "lightning strike" events during my childhood to initiate these perceptions, but perhaps I should revise my statement. The weather actually played an important role in deepening my awareness of the thought atmosphere. Although weather is a common occurrence throughout the world, the characteristics of weather vary greatly depending on the region. Weather patterns demonstrate a variety of behavior or traits—the coming together of clouds, rainfall, snow, hail, strong winds, soft breezes, high or low pressure changes, increases or decreases in temperature, electrical discharges, and so on. Where you live in the world determines the kinds of weather you are familiar with and, subsequently, the kind of distinctions you have learned to make about the weather.

For example, during the summer months in the Midwest, ominous weather patterns pay their regular visits. Growing up in the Chicago area, I learned to make distinctions about the weather based on certain indications. I noticed that when the color of the sky grew a dark hue of blue, it was going to be a garden-variety thunderstorm, strong winds with rain and lightning, but the storm activity would be far from our home or pass through with minimal destruction. These storms were not much cause for alarm, and my brothers and sister and I often enjoyed watching the spidery display of lights in the distant sky.

However, when weather of phenomenal force was gathering nearby, the indications were much different. I watched as the birds and squirrels took refuge well before there were any indications in the sky. Soon after, the air stood still, warm, thick, and heavy. When the color of the sky turned from dark blue to seaweed green that meant very destructive weather was approaching, and the neighborhood fled to their basements for safety. During storms of this magnitude, tornados would form or lightning struck the ground near our home. On one occasion, lightning struck our neighbor's house, and it caught fire. As strange as this may sound, you can learn a lot about lightning when it strikes within a hundred feet of where you are standing, *if* you pay close attention.

For me, the weather was more than a show of natural force. It was an opportunity to connect with the palpable unseen elements of the atmosphere. Since electrical storms occurred with seasonal regularity, I could track my senses along with the stimulation of the atmosphere during each electrical episode. A few moments before lightning made contact with the ground near my vicinity, I could detect physical variations in the air around me.

Many people are familiar with the experience of static electricity. The daily acts of combing hair or walking across the carpet and then brushing against an object can create the sparking sensation that we all know. When the electrons in the atmosphere build an electrical charge from this activity or stimulus, they eventually reach a crescendo and discharge. Static electricity discharges, for all practical purposes, are lightning strikes on a much smaller scale.

When lighting strikes, the ordinary household experience of static electricity is dramatically increased. Not only did the hair on my head rise, but so did every hair follicle on my body. I felt as if I was a human pin cushion, and at the same time, I felt as if I was a hot air balloon rising. The atmospheric draw on my hair was so strong it was as though I was being pulled off the ground. I also heard a "popping" or "clicking" sound similar to the sound you hear from a static discharge, but no sparks were observed. I also had my first experience with the flavor of electricity. A metallic taste occurred in my mouth moments before the lightning made contact with the earth. My body awareness went beyond the local field where the surface of my skin makes contact with the air and exceeded my arm's reach. I could feel the atmosphere next to my skin, and at the same time, I could feel the atmosphere on the other side of the room. Somehow, I was connected to the chain of air molecules all around me, and the orchestration of my senses reached a crescendo when the lightning flashed and discharged.

A few minutes later, the process repeated as electrical charges gathered and released during the thunderstorm. Once the lightning struck, the experience did not end instantly either. There was a gradual relaxation of the atmosphere around me until the air returned to its usual feeling. Learning about sensory perceptions from lightning strikes can be tricky because the event happens very quickly. You must make as many distinctions about your experience as possible in a very short amount of time. Your sensory channels move quickly through a cycle of low-level sensation to high-level sensation and return to low-level sensation in a fraction of a moment. If you do not recognize the cycle as it happens, then you simply perceive it as a single bursting sensation. There were not many other sensory experiences that illuminated my senses with such magnitude; sight, sound, touch, taste, and smell all occurring in a five-part harmony.

The dark olive skies did not come as often as I wanted, but when lightning storms occurred, I devoted my entire consciousness to the event. I stopped whatever I was doing so my five senses could scout and retrieve from their individual territories. With each passing experience, I opened more dimensions of perception. I also set perceptual markers to establish a range of sensory activity. One marker was when the atmosphere was at rest, such as a calm sunny day with little weather activity. The other was when the atmosphere was tense such as agitation in the air due to electrical storms. With these two markers in place, I moved back and forth with my perception by noticing the difference between high and low levels of atmospheric activity. I became increasingly aware of the behavior of the atmosphere around me at all times, not only during storms. When the atmosphere is stimulated to the degree that it produces a lightning strike is when most people pay attention to the effects. No one really pays attention to the molecular activity of the atmosphere during calm and sunny weather, we simply appreciate the beautiful day.

However, the molecules of the air are always in a state of stimulation, whether a storm is occurring or not, and opportunities abound to become sensitive to their activity. Human beings tend to live in areas where weather patterns are calm, and raging storms are the exception. Since atmospheric calm is where we spend most of our perceptual time, it is a powerful place to increase awareness since it is largely uninvestigated. This may sound utterly ridiculous, but I recognized that slowing down, separating, and identifying the individual stages of this quickly moving perceptual experience of molecular activity could be usefully applied.

Eventually, I noticed that *any* given moment, every environment, has a tactile level of atmospheric activity that contains a detectable level of sensation. With this awareness in place, I noticed how the atmosphere became influenced by human activities. Have you ever had the experience of entering a room when two people are having or have just completed an argument and noticed something in the air? Although the people in the room may appear to be calm and relaxed, there is a "tension" or "agitation" in the air that tells you all was not peaceful prior to your entrance. Have you ever stopped to wonder what it is that you are detecting?

Once again, I took the experience one step further, and I remained in place whenever I encountered people in arguments. I noticed how the charge of the room moved through an increasing and decreasing pattern of intensities during controversy and the residual effects thereafter. The atmosphere seemed to have its own microweather stimulated by the emotional and intellectual expressions of the people engaged in the argument. I could feel that the vibration of thoughts and emotions infused the spoken word and stimulated the molecules in the atmosphere. The idea of a microlightning storm occurring around you during your interactions may also sound ridiculous, but paying close attention to the atmospheric stimulation during emotional discharges allowed me to develop this kind of awareness. Through an everyday event known as disagreement, I began to learn about the raised "vibrational" alphabetical characters of the thought atmosphere. Since I can not see the molecules of air, I learned to translate what I could feel in the air; I taught myself atmospheric Braille.

I moved into my adolescence with this newfound perspective. As a result, I paid more attention to the ways people influenced the atmosphere around them. Eventually, I became curious to know how *I* affected the atmosphere around *me*. I learned about its textural qualities. It felt as a private universe in my circumference; a cloud of free-floating microstars that contained my memories, past, present, and future, as well as information about my personality, my emotions, my thoughts, and ideas.

Like many children, as I grew up, I began to contest authority. As turbulent as youth can sometimes be, these moments of angst provided me with unique opportunities to learn about the thought atmosphere. Whenever I engaged in verbal disagreements with my parents and peers, I noticed new kinds of body sensations emerging and competing for my attention over the thought atmosphere. These sensations included rushes of adrenaline, increases in body temperature or perspiration, my heart pounding in my chest, butterflies in my stomach, dryness and tension in my throat area, and so on. When we experience any one of these body sensations, or the combination thereof, it is commonly referred to as being nervous. Many people have an experience of these kinds of body sensations when speaking publicly in front of a large group of people.

Intense body sensations can be distracting during any conversations. However, I noticed that the higher the personal stakes are in a conversation, the greater the likelihood that these kinds of body sensations will occur. There were times when these body sensations interfered with my conversations so greatly that I was at a loss for words. I could not participate effectively during very important discussions. Again, I took the experience one step further, and during periods of conflict, I did what I could to resist the body sensations and stay focused on the thought atmosphere. But I was unsuccessful; in fact, the body sensations always prevailed. I wondered why the human body would have a built-in communication system to warn and empower us about our health, and at the same time, have a built-in "nervousness" mechanism that would disempower our personal communication.

I probably would not have lent any attention to the idea of a thought atmosphere had it not been for my early experiences with lightning storms. If you have not had the experience of being close to lighting when it strikes, that is okay—you do not have to chase thunderstorms in order to access the micro behavior of the air. You can have the experience of atmospheric activity in the safety of your own home.

Prominent Points for Chapter Review

- The indicators have the ability to detect an illness in its developmental stages. This feature makes it a powerful adjunct to conventional medical early detection methods.

- Opportunities to increase your sensory awareness are everywhere: thunderstorms, baseball games, shopping at the mall, etc.

- Develop a practice of paying attention to the distinctions you can perceive in the atmosphere as you go about your daily activities.

Practical Application

If you would like to have your own experience of the stimulation of the atmosphere, here are a few tips I can share.

- Lie down and get in a relaxed position.

- Set lights to a comfortable level for you.

- Make sure your environment provides silence. Do not play music, sound tones, or any other relaxation inducing stimulus. Make sure all televisions and radios are turned off. You want as little noise as possible.

- Focus on your breathing as you relax.

- Bring your awareness to your sense of hearing. Notice what you hear while you listen to the sound of a quiet room.

- After a while, you will likely notice that a quiet room is not soundless. Can you hear a soft hissing, whooshing, or a sound similar to when you place a seashell against your ear? This sound is distinct from a ringing in the ear.

- I call this noise the sound of air. Focus your auditory sense until you become aware of this sound.

- Maintain your audible connection with the ambient sound of air as you move into deeper relaxation. But avoid falling asleep; you need to come as close to sleep as you can without falling asleep.

- Once you are relaxed and can hear the soft audible sensation, focus completely on the sound. At some point, the volume should naturally increase on its own when you achieve this connection. Since you have become more sensitive to your sense of hearing, the sound can become loud. You may also hear static discharges, "popping," or "crunching" sounds (what I call walking on cornflakes).

- Notice what other forms of perception come forth during this event. The hair on your body may become very sensitive to atmospheric stimuli or even stand on end. You may *feel* other body sensations during this event. It may take some practice until you have the experience that I have described.

CHAPTER NINE

Discourse, Dialogue, and Decisions

A S I CONTINUED to jump through the hoops of science at the Bethesda medical office, some of my earlier decisions about the indicators were up for reinterpretation. I wanted to know what it meant if a person had a conventional diagnosis of illness, but no indicators were present. Until now, when someone told me they had been diagnosed with a disease, and I had not observed an indicator, my conclusion was that medical science must be correct, and the indicators were off target. A confirmed conventional diagnosis had always been the measure of truth, but as I reviewed my past, the indicators seemed to have been on target all along. I inquired more often with friends and colleagues who had received a medical diagnosis but did not project any indicators to test my theory. Some of the people that I spoke to found that the conventional medical information they received was not only inaccurate but also very costly. I heard of unnecessary or questionable medical procedures and treatments that left people without answers and sometimes left people without body organs.

Polly was on the verge of tears when she told me her doctors had ordered the tests for leukemia. This was not a precaution, she said. Her physicians were certain, and the tests were a formality for insurance reasons. When I looked at Polly, she did not have the indicator of those I have seen with diseases of the blood. She was not losing moisture either. In fact, she did not demonstrate an indicator of any real consequence that I could determine; perhaps some mild indicators, but certainly no cause for alarm. A few months later, I saw her again and she was all smiles. Her tests for leukemia came back negative. It turned out to be nothing more than food allergies. I do not know how the doctors had made the leap from allergies to leukemia, but I am sure they had their reasons. I do know that the long period of leukemia tests, waiting for results, telling her friends and relatives of the impending doom, and follow-up visits with her physicians was an unnecessarily painful time for Polly and her family.

My friend Bonnie had been told by her physicians that she would not be able to conceive children because she was infertile. She and her husband were devastated by the news because having a child was their greatest desire. However, when I looked at her, I saw no indicator of infertility. It seemed to me that her physician's evaluation, compounded with their upset about not being able to conceive a child, was interfering with their reproductive process more than any biological malfunctions. She insisted on artificial insemination although her physician told her that it would be a waste of time and money. Bonnie's dreams of being a mother grew dim.

The next time I saw Bonnie, a few years had passed, but she was not alone. Bonnie had given birth to a beautiful baby girl.

Sherry Anne told me her physician wanted to pursue a series of tests for a suspected cardiovascular problem. They had recommended that she undergo a rather invasive testing procedure called a thallium stress test. The way this test works is by injecting a radioactive dye into the cardiovascular system, and the dye allows a device to observe the contractions of the heart.

Sherry Anne felt there was nothing wrong with her cardiovascular system and that the test was unnecessary and a waste of time and money. She wanted another opinion, and she met with me to evaluate her indicators. I told her that I did not observe a cardiovascular indicator when I looked at her. Sherry Anne returned to her physicians and advocated for another approach to testing her cardiovascular system. A cardiac workup was performed, and no abnormalities were found. The radioactive test was cancelled.

Likewise, it had been several years since I last saw Nelly. When we met again, she looked happy and healthy. We caught up on each other's lives, and during our conversations, she told me that her gall bladder had been surgically removed. Her words took me by surprise. When an organ or system has fallen into such decay that it needs to be removed, it often leaves an indicator scar even if removal has restored the body to health. She looked full of moisture to me, and I did not detect even the slightest scar of a gall bladder indicator. Before I could drop my jaw and show my surprise, she quickly said, "The funny thing was that when the doctors removed my gall bladder and actually looked at the organ, there was nothing diseased about it. It was pink and healthy—oops!" After the surgery, her doctors suggested they may have been mistaken about the gall bladder but told

Nelly they were certain that the removal of another body organ might be a good idea. After losing her gall bladder for no reason, she was reluctant to sacrifice another piece of her anatomy for the sake of troubleshooting. Nelly's response to her physicians was, "Thanks, but no thanks." Her health has remained intact ever since.

It became abundantly clear that the body's model of indicators has its own voice and needs to "stand as its own" health assessment process. This is not to be confused with a "stand alone" health assessment model. If the information presented by the indicators is contrary to a conventional diagnosis, rather than quickly defaulting to medical science, further testing should be performed to identify why these inconsistencies exist and hold both assessment models with equal weight. I kept in contact with anyone I knew who had a confirmed medical diagnosis and did not demonstrate any indicators for more evidence.

When the study first began, I wanted to get the highest score of accuracy possible, so I *only* reported the indicators that I saw. I realized now that was a mistake because the information I withheld turned out to be relevant to the patient's path of recovery. I needed to widen my aperture of understanding and find out what the body was truly saying and fully activate this universal language of health. I knew the meaning of my perceptions exceeded the description I gave Len and Beth on the first day in their office, but at the time, I decided to present my explanations in a rational way with editorial diplomacy. Otherwise, it might have been misinterpreted as flowery rhetoric. Since the study had a firm foundation at this juncture, I decided to report all that I perceived and share with Beth the discretionary information I had withheld, even if that meant pushing the envelope.

Patient 14013: "Elizabeth"

John: She has a second-degree respiratory indicator and a first-degree gastrointestinal indicator.

Beth: She has been diagnosed with asthma and allergic rhinitis. I wonder if the gastrointestinal indicator corresponds to the vague right upper quadrant abdominal pain that she has had on and off for years. Interestingly enough, all conventional medical tests of her intestines to date . . . have turned up negative.

John: That's because her digestive system doesn't know about her asthma.

Beth: I'm not sure what you mean. What does her digestive system have to do with her asthma?

John: We both agree that all of the body organs and systems are related to one another—not just related, but affected by one another. Sometimes I have to find the best words to explain information, so let me think out loud for a few minutes. The human body is a unified, integrated, and interrelated system. What happens to one organ affects the balance of the whole system. Not only that, but each organ has consciousness and is able to perceive and be aware of changes in the other organs as well. So what I am saying is that there is a breakdown in communication between her organs. Her digestive system doesn't know about her asthma.

Beth: How do you know?

John: Because her lungs just told me.

Beth: Come again?

John: Beth, there's a lot I haven't told you.

Beth: Okay, I am listening. So you are saying that body organs talk to one another and to you?

John: Well . . . yes, but again, this communication is available through the ordinary senses. It's not magic. But this is something I am telling you for the first time. The body . . . has a natural capacity for what I call . . . intraorgan communication.

Beth: Really? Explain that to me.

John: Think of the human body as a corporation. There are different departments such as finance, accounting, marketing, and so on. The success of the corporation relies heavily on the quality of communication between the interdependent departments. In terms of metabolic activities, the human body operates much the same way.

Sometimes, however, the communication breaks down, and that's when the corporation is in financial or operational jeopardy. There can be several causes for this breakdown in body communication, but some of the primary ones are when people feel they have lost command of their lives. They are just along for the ride of circumstances. Depressed psychological states can also bring about breakdown. Another cause is when people disconnect from their emotions so deeply and live solely from intellect that they have the experience of becoming disconnected from their body. Add lethargy, or the lack of physical activity to the mix, and it can make for poor levels of intraorgan communication. In general, people's organs interact within the body's biological community with varying degrees of efficiency. I use a percentage scale to evaluate the quality of this communication. Like the moisture level, an average healthy range of communication is 80-100 percent. Unlike the moisture level, the intraorgan communication level can drop to a low level without allowing the system to be overcome by illness. Low levels of communication correlate to a sluggish or depressed state of organ functionality. If a person has an indicator present and their level of intraorgan communication is below 80 percent, the effect of the imbalance is compounded. The return to health becomes much more challenging, not to mention that their daily experience of life is probably a miserable one. Even worse, if an indicator is present, a low level of communication exists, *and* they are also losing moisture, the prognosis becomes rather bleak.

Beth: Exactly how do you access this intraorgan communication?

John: It's very simple, but *simple* seems to be a very relative term in this study.

Beth: So it's simple for you, but maybe not for others. Are you saying that you hear voices?

John: No. It is another kind of language; one of vibration. We are getting into a new realm of awareness or what I call *textures of consciousness*. The individual body organs and systems are cognizant of our own thoughts. They are also cognizant of our personalities, our feelings, our memories . . . Basically they are aware of our comprehensive life experience. Recall our earlier conversation when I said that 'thought has sound,' and 'sound has form.' This kind of organ communication is accessed by blending the senses, but not in the same way as when I look at indicators. I take it one step further. When I combine my sense of hearing with my already combined sense of sight and touch, another sense emerges, and I can *hear* with my eyes. It is not mind reading because if you are thinking about who won the football game last night or your favorite color, those kinds of thoughts are not important to the body organs and do not register in the thought atmosphere, nor does it convey any information to me. The thought atmosphere does not lend attention to trivial data. It's about identity. However, I can hear how people put their thoughts together, how they assemble their cognition and their emotions, if that makes any sense to you at all. I don't *hear* any sounds, but ideas can be felt as they are assembled into statements of meaning. Do you remember when we were at the mall and I mentioned electrical telepathy—bits of data flying all around us in a binary code, ones and zeros, that can be translated into words and meaning? Like indicators, people project their own thought code. I am very familiar with the set of ones and zeros in my own thought atmosphere. Whenever I want to engage intraorgan communication, I allow other people's binary code to interface with mine. When people project their code at me and the two codes meet, mine and theirs, I can translate their data using my own binary code as a primer. Since I already know many of the words generated in my own thought atmosphere, based on my own content, I know how to assemble the words and meanings of others by using my own code. The best way I can describe this experience is a felt series of pulsations that emit from people, but I also *feel* with my *ears* as I *look* at a person. When all three senses are engaged simultaneously, I enter another multiperceptual mode. Since I know how to perceive the pulsation interval and rate, I convert this "vibrating" content into words and sentences. The thought atmosphere is interactive, and a "ping" will generate a prompt for information. Our bodies naturally communicate which creates a call and response, and because there is so much information contained in the code, detecting the language through the atmosphere is fairly simple to do once you are in this blended sensory state.

Beth: Do you walk around hearing what's going on with people?

John: At first, people's thought encodings bombarded me. I couldn't stop from hearing it or escape the noise. Highly populated places such as airports or subways were extremely difficult for me. In crowded places, people's internal conversations are flying all over the place unconsciously. It was especially offensive when their thoughts were full of negative or unkind content. Since people broadcast themselves, my tendency was to listen because I didn't know how to turn the volume down or off. In time, I learned how to regulate or repel people's projected communications on an individual basis. Eventually, public places or social settings with large groups of people became easier for me. Now, I am only as affected as I want to be. People often ask me how I hear what is going on with other people. I laugh because, believe it or not, people are careless with their projections, it's the other way around, I had to learn how *not* to hear.

Beth: I can understand on an intellectual level what you are saying and how this might be possible . . . but I still can't begin to understand *how* you do it even after you just told me all that.

John: Let me explain in another way. The thought atmosphere is meshed with the body. When people project their thoughts to me, I feel it in the atmosphere around them and around me *and* within me. It is much the same as striking a tuning fork that stimulates other metals nearby, causing them to vibrate. My body has become an instrument, like a harp. Whenever I am in the presence of another person, their radiant thoughts and emotions cause certain stimulations of the atmosphere around me, which then plays certain strings within me. When I was younger, I learned to connect certain feelings in the air around me to certain strings within me. The way I identified which words were connected to which strings was based on the regularity of a string played within me and what was occurring. The situation I was in had a lot to do with determining which word or words groups I assembled by the plucking of the different strings within me. At first, I only had a few strings, ten or twelve, but over time, I developed hundreds of strings that created a rather full vocabulary for me. The ability to understand the thought atmosphere communication can be useful for revealing the details behind a person's health imbalance. Not details in the scientific sense of raised enzyme levels or vitamin deficiencies, but those of the human element, details that include personality and emotional distresses behind the body organ or system breakdown. Now that you mention it, it *does* become a voice in a round about way. What I see is not science, which is probably why there are some discrepancies between indicators and conventional medical diagnosis. What I see is a language of health . . . the body's visible language.

Beth: So what else can you do with this visible language?

John: That is a very big question. Are you ready to cross the Rubicon?

Beth: Ha! Okay, go ahead!

John: Identifying a distressed body organ or system is only one of its uses. It can also be used to create a *comprehensive* health assessment, bringing forth the messages sequestered within the body. As we have said before, there is no way to accurately measure whether or not a person is living a self-examined life. If people have difficulty identifying the blind spots in their life, then this information can accelerate the process of self-awareness and reveal the underlying content. As we both agree, uncovering those messages is integral to the process of healing. But as we have talked about already, some people don't like the messages they receive. Again, much depends on whether or not a person is willing to hear what their body has to say about their life. I already have some experience with how people handle receiving personal information. It can evoke quite a bit of upset or denial. Sometimes the messages from the body confront their lifestyles, behaviors, attitudes, and beliefs about their life. For many people, these aspects of their life are not up for negotiation or concession, but often, when people are experiencing a health crisis, this is where the answers can be found. There is more going on with people's health than just what can be observed under the microscope. Dialogue with the body organs and systems has the potential to cut to the proverbial chase. When *all* the information about their body system is revealed and presented to the patient, they can approach their path of healing fully prepared, clearly aware, and empowered. Searching the blind spots discloses much of the underlying directives that promote the breakdown of health. It can reveal the origins of physical ailments that have been the cause of pain and suffering for long periods of time. For this reason, it is at least as important as identifying indicators. What I am telling you isn't news. The mind-spirit-body connection concept has been around for a long time. But if people can allow this information to come through, it offers people the opportunity to deeply examine their lives so that they can begin to unravel the messages from within. I am not convinced that illness is some kind of lesson or a punitive lash from our bodies due to neglect of the information it sends. My sense is that anatomy or physiology is the only language the body knows how to speak, and it certainly has one very effective way of getting our attention—by throwing a biological tantrum through illness. The symptoms that surface in the body are interwoven with clues from the body that can lead to healing, but symptoms are not necessarily a separate source of medical information in and of themselves.

Beth: Okay, so that being said, what kind of effect does the breakdown of communication between this patient's respiratory and digestive systems have on her health?

I explained to Beth that our research was about to exceed the domain of scientific medicine.

John: Throughout the clinical trials we have tried to fit these indicators into the mold of conventional medicine. In this study, by design, my perceptions must meet and satisfy protocols of reliability, validity, and reproducibility because according to scientific methods used in medicine, everything must be verifiable in order to be legitimate. Any new claims or ideas must be pushed through a mental mill and, ideally, flush out the mechanism that explains how it works. In order to validate this vocabulary of indicators, it must correlate to established and accepted scientific medical constructs. The problem, of course, is that my process of identifying health imbalances cannot be entirely explained. On one hand, this concerns me because evidence-based science requires an explanation. On the other hand, if we only embrace what the scientific process affirms as legitimate, we may be missing some of the most important gifts that human beings have to offer. I am not saying that we throw away logic and reason and replace them with fantasy. The value of the empirical process we have used in the study delivers the results science wants.

But it doesn't demonstrate the path to those results that science wants to see. I now wonder if the way we have structured this clinical study won't allow us to see the big picture either.

This technique of using the senses, by its own definition, extends beyond scientific borders. But my point here is that no single approach can fully explain all that we know. Some phenomena may not lend themselves to scientific rigor and statistical analysis at this point in time simply because we don't have the methods or devices sensitive enough to measure certain kinds of phenomena. But that does not mean that techniques that cannot be explained are not valid. We still haven't found the mechanism that is responsible for gravity. Scientists have some ideas and have identified some of the elements, but if we truly knew what that mechanism is . . . we could play with gravity . . . alter the effects of gravity.

But come to think of it, in the past, science hasn't been available to embrace many new ideas no matter how logical they have been. Even those anointed within the field of medicine with brilliant new practical approaches—scientists such as Joseph Lister—encountered huge opposition. In the early days of surgery, medical science would not recognize the important correlation between the sterilized hands of the surgeons and the occurrence of postsurgical infections. The empirical evidence was present. People died unnecessarily from infection after surgery even though the surgery itself was a success. It was the cause, or mechanism, of the infection that was mysterious, and the debate surrounding the explanation raised quite a controversy in the medical community. When one doctor came forward and advocated simply washing hands before performing an operation, he was considered a boat-rocking renegade troublemaker by medical science. It took a long time, even with solid reproducible evidence, to ease the collective mind of medical science and gradually recognize that post surgical infection is most often due to the lack of sterilization procedures. Now, the required procedure prior to surgery is sterilizing the hands and instruments. Today, there are far less postsurgical infections as a result.

Beth: Well, yes. Quite often, intellectual musings and theories must come before scientific proof. Theory and practice are a cycle. Practice produces information and problems, which leads to theory, which leads to testing in practice.

John: But at the fundamental level, you and I have been seeking the mechanism that allows these perceptions of health in order to gain the attention of medical science. If we rely solely on logic, reason, and scientific principles, we can only go so far. If we want to cross the bridge between what we know about health and healing and what we do not know, then where we go from here may not have an observable mechanism given the current understandings of science, only measurable results, like gravity. There is no conventional medical test to determine if a person is authentically investigating the blind spots of their lives. Subsequently, organ messages are not quantifiable or measurable either. However, it is confirmable nonetheless because there is evidence through one important mechanism that *is* available to us: patient feedback. So how do you want to proceed with the study? Do you want to keep on making sure that the indicators fit nicely into the boxes of medical science, or do you want to stand on the plateau of body perception and look beyond?

Beth: I am open to expanding the scope of the study. I am really curious to see where this is all going, but at the same time the information . . . the applications . . . they still need to be relevant to our scientific medical assessment and procedures. If you can use this organ communication to tell me something I don't already know medically as a clinician, then it's useful, but if it comes across as "incense and crystals," don't expect to get very far with the conventional medical community even if what you are saying is critically important.

John: Fair enough. So back to the patient we were discussing. Let's see what I can offer you. Depending on the severity of her asthma, the effects will vary. It seems to me that logically, if her blood does not receive the required amount of oxygen to perform the necessary functions of all the body systems, then the effects could be widespread. Specific to her condition, if the digestive system does not have the optimal level of oxygen to carry out the function of digestion, let's postulate that there is a possibility that the process of digestion could be compromised or labored because of the reduced oxygen level. I'll take another leap here, and correct me if I am inaccurate, but I assume that when someone seeks health care because they are experiencing digestive complaints, a health care provider would not typically investigate the respiratory systems as a way to understanding the digestive system.

Beth: No. Not generally speaking.

John: You already know what happened with Rhonda and how her ophthalmologist didn't see the connection between her eyes and her thyroid. I am assuming that medical science would also consider the respiratory system and asthma to be mutually exclusive from the breakdown of the digestive system.

Beth: Yes.

John: So let's explore this possibility of how her asthma might relate to her vague abdominal complaints. Remember, we are talking about the relationship between the body organs and systems. We already talked about the body resembling a corporation. But we must think beyond a profit-maximizing scheme. We must wear the suit of a biological corporation that includes the mental, emotional, and spiritual aspect of being. These aspects of being are often excluded in our corporate business climate today, and it's no wonder why people lack fulfillment in the workplace, but I'm getting off topic now.

Beth: This is not new. Really, the study of human physiology has always been based on systems theory. This just takes it to the next level—the human body as a system that interacts and is modified by the mind and the spirit. It also relates to the burgeoning science of psychoneuroimmunology, whose main postulate is that the nerve fibers that carry emotions, pain, and immune functions all modulate each other. This whole scientific branch was started by mistake in a laboratory by a gentleman by the name of Robert Ader in the 1970s. Another pioneer in this area has been Candace Pert, who discovered that the cells responsible for emotion are located in every cell of the body, not just the brain. She also noted that unexpressed emotions are stored in these cells and create a hidden vault of information that may eventually be expressed as illness in the body. In her book, *Molecules of Emotion*, she goes on to discuss how emotions are the nexus between the mind and matter and that they move back and forth between the two, influencing both, part of a system where each part communicates with the others. Now that I think of it, there is another pocket of science that theorizes the presence of subatomic particles that scientists are unsure how to classify. One moment they behave as matter and the next they behave as energy. The theory goes on to suggest that perhaps they are both at the same time. Perhaps this vibrational stimulus that you keep talking about and/or Candace Pert's molecules of emotions is actually related to the fluctuation between the two states of matter and energy. You have said that people's bodies *project* indicators, so perhaps your perception could relate to emissions at the subatomic level.

One of the reasons that this whole project is so interesting to me is that pieces of your perceptual abilities can be correlated to what these cutting-edge scientists are discovering in other venues. So in your model, what causes this communication breakdown between the organs? Why doesn't the body remain in open communication with itself on all levels at all times?

John: Another great question . . . This answer is a little more complex.

Beth: I had a feeling it might be.

John: This language of vibration can provide much more information than just telling me that two organs are not on speaking terms. As I have worked with these perceptions over my lifetime, I have noticed that the body is a reflection of what is occurring in our lives. The reflections contain both obscure and straightforward information. Quite often, what happens is the body will send us messages alerting us to areas in our life where we are underperforming or undervaluing our own path of development.

Beth: You mean our symptoms alert us when we are not performing our spiritual tasks?

John: That's almost it. When you speak of spiritual tasks or the meaning of life, each person's journey will be unique. Our learning can come from many different directions. The six billion or so people on earth today all have a mélange of living agendas, if you will, challenges and triumphs, gains and losses to experience. The common denominator for all people in the face of such a rich experiential mix is a physical body. The body is the one consistent element among all people. It is the one true decoder ring.

Beth: Okay, so what I am hearing you say is that the human body is an instrument, a vehicle that we as human beings use to act out our spiritual tasks. The messages that the body produces maintain a consistent theme. What's more, the reason people experience persistent health conditions is they do not *allow* the illness to deliver its message and expose the theme.

John: Ah, but take the next step. And look further, our bodies are not just a biological vehicle we use to get around on the planet. What if our bodies actually have a conscious stake in our life's journey? What if it actually matters to our bodies whether or not we succeed at exposing the theme?

Beth: So applying that idea to this patient, for whatever reason, this patient's asthma persists because the underlying message is not being heard. People's symptoms are their spiritual tasks. Her asthma persists *because* she is not able to hear what her respiratory system has to say—the task remains undone!

John: Exactly. Examples of underperforming or undervaluing can include giving ourselves away, engaging in self-defeating behavior, hiding our light and power, lack of boundaries, and so on. My words probably sound like jargon. Remember, I have a leadership seminar background, but they are fairly accurate descriptions of what people do when they sabotage themselves. Awareness is the first step. If you don't know that you are sabotaging yourself, there is little room for improvements. Depending on which body organ or system is acting out tells me more about the nature of the message. I am not the first to bring these ideas forward. It's the old chili in a new can, but what I have noticed missing in professional health circles, both conventional or alternative, is that no one has given the body its own voice. Conventional medicine doesn't *ask* the body tissues on the slides under the microscope what is going on. Many of the ancient medical traditions were influenced by the social values of the time. While these traditions hold many truths, the body's natural language of health is diachronic. Much has changed over the centuries, and the social values of the times that influenced older traditions and rituals may no longer connect with the requirements of our modern era. For example, many years ago, individual records or personal information accounts were maintained for only certain members of society, such as royalty or priests. No records were kept for an individual citizen. Nowadays, private information accounts are maintained for almost everyone. Financial information and spending behaviors are monitored and influenced by several mediums that have effects on the ways people live. Our individual needs are much more complex now, and our daily activities are vastly different from what they were a few thousand years ago. These changes in activities have evolved into new social demands and, subsequently, new demands for the human mind and body. An evolution of the mind-body-spirit connection has occurred and will continue to occur so long as we exist. I am using this technique to identify where and how these evolutionary variables have linked information with the body's maladies.

Beth: Are we talking about karma?

John: I don't think so. I am talking about our DNA having an encoding, an embedded blueprint that links messages to maladies to organs to indicators as a possible explanation for this phenomenology. It is this evolutionary blueprint that also bonds us as a species.

Beth: So what you're saying is that we need to identify a reliable and consistent source of health information that pertains to our modern society. The body is that source because it provides feedback to each individual as they pursue their respective life journeys. This feedback is invaluable as it provides insight into the cycle of health, illness, and vitality. It helps to clarify the connection between organ system dysfunction, emotions, and life experiences. This is confirming for me because it so clearly connects to my work as a transpersonal therapist. I use Gestalt therapy and a variety of other techniques to help people use their life experiences, emotions, and dreams to reveal and understand obstacles they encounter along the way. I have found that there are basic themes in peoples' life experiences (and emotions and dreams) that tend to repeat over and over again, sometimes literally, often metaphorically. Furthermore, these metaphoric stories set the meter or tone for a person's life. This sounds very similar to what you were saying before about the body producing a consistent theme. I have observed that it seems to be our job, our spiritual mission, to repeat these stories or themes over and over again until we truly understand the underlying message. Hmm, I wonder if what sets the meter or tone that correlates to the body organ systems is the same information you get from your visual perception technique.

John: As I have dialogued with people's bodies over the years—

Beth: Wait a minute; you said *dialogue*. That's more than just listening! You can talk *back* to the organs?

John: Well . . . I said this was going to be a stretch. Remember, we are looking beyond the borders of science. I already told you how I convert information from the body into words. Thought has sound and sound has form. Whenever I want additional information or clarity from the body, all I need do is think of the question I want to ask. The sound of the question in my mind takes form in my thought atmosphere. My atmosphere then assembles and sends its own encoded message that the thought atmosphere of the other person can decode, and then their thought atmosphere formulates a vibrational reply. Again, it's basically call and response that we are talking about here. I take a piece of clay and mold it, then hand it to you. You reshape it and hand it back to me.

Beth: I am still not clear about how this is done.

John: Well, I don't know how to build an engine, but I do know how to drive a car.

Beth: Let's get back to life and how it relates to organ dysfunction.

John: I have encountered consistent messages that the *body* has assigned to each of the organs or systems because of what the *body* has told me. There are no absolutes here. There are details to sort, some variations to recognize since individual experiences will vary, but the themes are general. Some of my information may parallel meanings and interpretations made within other traditions, but many do not. These themes are not my ideas either. I am simply reporting what the body has told me.

Beth: What is the respiratory message for this patient?

John: If she were still here, I could show you how the dialogue process works. But generally speaking, the respiratory system often points to "perceived injustice."

Beth: Interestingly enough . . . I have done several Gestalt sessions with her, and I can say that based on what I know . . . your assessment is accurate.

John: The reason I say "perceived" is because much of our reality is determined from our own point of view. Two people can have the same experience and interpret the event in two entirely different manners. Somewhere along the way, an event (or series of events) has occurred for this woman that she has interpreted life to be unjust. Although she may experience grief, anger, or upset, these are not interpretations. These are emotions that result from the interpretation. When someone experiences an event that disconnects them from harmony or happiness, the workings of the mind collect all the data from the experience: who was involved, what emotions came forward, what was said, what actions were taken, what elements of reality or beliefs were reinforced, how the event resolved, and so on. The person gathers these *perceptual* components and then moves them through their inner filters, world view, belief systems, whatever you want to call it, until they arrive at a judgment or conclusion about the experience. Depending upon which interpretations they arrive at will determine which organ becomes activated. In effect, the person processes the experience and the interpretation activates the corresponding body systems. Yes, the body holds emotions, but the organs hold explanations.

People often fail to recognize that they are *perceiving* life through filters. Instead, they think life *is* real—it *is* the way it *is*. Their interpretations of experience are factual for them and subsequently construct their realities. Patterns of behavior become coupled to the interpretations, and the basic ingredients are in place for the deterioration of health. Eventually, the constructs of reality and the patterns of behavior become frozen in place by our interpretations. If we can remember that we are selective about the ways we interpret our lives, then we have free will, then reality has choices. It becomes negotiable. But be careful. There is a huge difference between unfreezing patterns of behavior and constructs of reality and just changing your mind about life. If we just change our minds, then our interpretations may have us just take another trip around the block only to arrive at another detrimental interpretation and decision. That's because the limiting patterns and constructs of reality are still in place, and while you may correct one health imbalance, it will simply move to another area of the body and reactivate in another organ. I am sure you have heard of instances when a patient's ailment has been corrected by medical procedures, but then a new one surfaces somewhere else in the body. The root cause has not been addressed.

Beth: I can confirm that during clinical trials for developing new drugs or treatments, a similar event occurs. Let's say the test results showed that 80 percent of patients who took a new drug experienced decreased symptoms, relief, or even a cure. Everybody thinks that's wonderful success. The medical report says the drug works. But quite often, they don't tell us in the report that those participating in the study began having symptoms or discomforts manifest in other areas of the body that are unrelated to possible side effects of the medication.

John: Yes, simply treating the organ doesn't mean that the limiting patterns of belief or behaviors are removed. If this woman had interpreted from the event (or events) that she has no self-worth that leads to self-loathing, then the organ affected would likely be her skin, not her lungs.

Beth: So self-loathing is related to the skin. Have you been able to correlate all the organ dysfunctions with their emotional causes?

John: I know some of them, but not all. I know cardiovascular, digestion, thyroid, respiratory, blood, breast, liver, and reproduction. I haven't been able to observe every possible health imbalance, which has always been a limitation in our study. I haven't worked with many people who have kidney problems, so I am not sure what interpretations affect the kidneys.

Beth: You are basically referring to psychoanalysis. Sigmund Freud offered a systematic explanation and treatment of neurosis.

John: I am aware that Freud and others have presented models that explain the developmental course after childhood trauma. But I am looking at this through an indicator lens. What's interesting to me is that two people can have the same experience, and because of how they choose to interpret events, the end result is that two different organs or systems go into breakdown. When I say that reality is negotiable, I am not saying that if we reinterpret our beliefs that we can overthrow the prevailing laws of the natural forces. Human beings can't walk through walls or fly through the air. We aren't operating our belief systems on that level yet, but perhaps one day we will. In the meantime, we are all subject to an aspect of reality called gravity that we cannot overcome. What I am talking about are the ways that interpretations develop our identities. For example, two children can grow up in the same household with domestic violence, yet they often develop two distinct patterns of behavior as a way of coping or even surviving. Once they reach adulthood, one sibling may become an alcoholic while the other a workaholic, but either one is an effective method for avoiding pain. Their health imbalances will likely develop in two different body organs. People often think that because two people have two different health problems, the causes must be completely unrelated or different variables, and that is not necessarily the case. If the childhood trauma or cause is domestic violence, which holds true for each child, in other words a constant, it is their interpretations that determine the variable. Again, it's not actually "real." It is perceived, just as anyone's *reality* is derived. Sometimes people are conscious of the event that resulted in the interpretations, but oftentimes, they are not. Furthermore, reinterpreting anger into jealousy won't produce much progress. If anyone wants to transform their health or life, not just change their mind, the place to begin is to realize that one's experience of an event is relative, and not fixed. If people can reinterpret the event from a neutral place with the intentions of arriving at a positive interpretation, then the body can move toward balance. Sometimes very painful experiences have tremendous value to offer our lives, but many people never get to open their gift.

Beth: So what would be empowering for this patient is if she reexplored her past and identified the unjust events. She could reinterpret the events and unfreeze the limiting patterns of behavior linked to that decision. With the intent and recognition that how the unjust events were perceived would probably have a profound affect on her health or, in this case, her respiratory system.

John: This doesn't mean that we allow abuse in our lives and then tell ourselves it's not real and, therefore, allow abuses to persist. Healthy boundaries are important to all people, but anytime you positively reinterpret a decision that causes you pain and separation, it will bring you closer to unity.

Beth: That's correct. In fact, that is the reason I trained to be a transpersonal therapist. I wanted to help people to clarify and rectify, if possible, the emotional and spiritual issues that caused their physical pain and suffering.

In that moment, our interests broadened significantly. We continued to test the indicators for accuracy, but from then on, Beth and I spent long hours looking for consistencies between organ imbalances and the conversations sequestered within each one of the body systems.

Shortly thereafter, the opportunity to test the accuracy of intraorgan communication came when a woman requested to meet with me. We met, and I identified seven problematic health conditions. She confirmed my assessment by sharing her health history and the seven conventional diagnoses she had already received. She was very pleased with accuracy of the assessment . . . so far. However, when I assessed her reproductive system as "not seeing any activity to speak of," she was awestruck! "I have fibroid tumors!" she erupted. The other seven hits were no longer meaningful, and she looked at me, incredulous. I reemphasized that I was interpreting the body's language—this is not MRI vision—and that her body was much more concerned about the other areas of her health that we had already discussed. But my words brought her no comfort, and a silent tension commenced.

I broke the silence by asking her if she experienced physical pain from the tumors, and she replied, "No." I asked her if she experienced any loss of quality of life from these tumors, and she replied, "No." I asked her if these tumors had been diagnosed as malignant, progressive, or in any way a threat to her system, and she replied, "No." She added, "There was only one occurrence of bleeding many years ago, which alerted my attention and caused me to seek medical attention." Otherwise, she had no signs or symptoms. In fact, she would not have known about her fibroid tumors had her physician not examined her following the bleeding episode. I reaffirmed that her body was telling me that the tumors were not a threat to her system. This information did not pacify her, and she continued to stare at me puzzlingly. Once again, I had come to the place in a session where my words were in conflict with the client's disposition. But this time, I moved through and opened the channels of organ communication.

Within a few moments, I began to perceive her body's message about the origin of her tumors. Her lower pelvic region communicated to me that approximately thirteen years ago, she had abandoned a most precious pearl (the way I perceive numbers in years with health histories is similar to the way I perceived numbers with the mathematical flash cards. I feel the numbers in the atmosphere around the body the same as the atmosphere around the cards.) The result of the experience was equally interruptive to her creative expression. I told her what her body told me. She confirmed that when she was younger, she showed early talent as a promising actress. Creative expression brought her tremendous joy, and because of her considerable flair, she had received scholarships to attend acting school. However, her parents wanted her to pursue a practical career in the judicial system. She was conflicted and had to choose between her creative desire and her parent's desires. She acquiesced and abandoned her path of acting and followed her parent's practical wishes. Her career became law, and her tumors manifested at that exact time thirteen years ago.

We discussed her feelings about her decision. As she spoke, the light of joy returned to her face as she reconnected with her lost passion for the performing arts. But I also noticed that she was experiencing a deep reconnection with her body and the message from within. In that moment, I realized that informing people about their health is similar to a weather report. It is simple abstract information until they have their own experience of hearing what their body has to say instead of me telling them. When the message comes alive and "real" for people is when their healing can begin. I told her that her body probably has much more to tell her. I told her to go home, lie down, become silent, and talk to her lower pelvis. Through dialogue with her own organ system, she might hear more of what her body wanted her to know.

The next day, she called and said that she asked her body some questions but did not feel that she received any answers. However, she was experiencing bleeding from her reproductive region, which had not happened in several years. In my estimation, whatever conversation occurred between her and her lower pelvic region, even though she did not feel she received any responses, had catalyzed her biology. Her body *was* responding, along with the evidence from her body tissues. She just didn't know how to interpret the communication. However, the preliminary step to renegotiating the decisions, and subsequently, the patterns of disease had begun.

If physicians knew how to properly apply the indicators during interactions with their patients, it would open up new frontiers in prognosis. What if a physician could tell their patients, "Yes, you have tumors, but don't worry. They are not significant because they pose no threat to your health."

From then on, organ dialogue became integral to my work. The feedback from people confirmed the accuracy of what their body organs had to say. Sometimes the body spoke in literal terms as was the case with the woman with the fibroid tumors, but oftentimes, the information was metaphoric. When the body relayed a metaphoric scenario during the communication process, the client and I explored the symbolic meaning in the scenario in order to arrive at a clear understanding. Some people listened to the message from their body and some did not, but I pressed on.

§ § §

Sixteen months had passed since the first day I walked into Len and Beth's office on that autumn afternoon in November. Len called a meeting for the three of us, and I figured it meant we would expand the study and begin clinical testing of the hypotheses Beth and I had considered. When I arrived at the office, I met Beth in the waiting room. She accompanied me to one of the examination rooms, and we sat down. Len walked in with a thick folder in his hand that held the compared assessments from the study and many of our notes. He set them on the table and sat down.

"John, you should be pleased with what you have accomplished."

"Thanks, Len, having access to your office, patients, and medical expertise, we know so much more about the indicators now although there is more to learn. I have developed two separate evaluation sheets, one for men and one for women, since Beth and I found that there are some indicator differences between the sexes" (see appendix E and F).

Beth added, "Yes, John, the past several months have been very interesting, and I am privileged to have worked on such a project. Few health care providers have the opportunity to explore medicine in their practice like we have."

"Thank you too, Beth. None of this would have been possible without your support either. I will always be grateful . . . but it sounds like you two are saying good-bye."

Len continued, "Beth tells me you are teaching her how to use this ability with her patients. That's an important piece!"

"Yes," I replied, "Beth and I have ideas about how to teach people to see their own health. In fact, we have so many ideas we really don't know where to begin. But isn't that why we are having this meeting . . . to discuss our next step?"

Len chuckled. "Be careful what you ask for, John. You just might get it."

"What do you mean?" I asked.

"John, you achieved what you set out to do. Your testing here in my office has provided the validation you were seeking that first day we met. You've convinced me anyway," Len added.

"Okay, but what happens now? Where do we go with the study next, Len?"

"Unfortunately, the research doesn't go much further here. You have assessed all the patients who were willing to participate in the study. I have afforded you all the office space and time that I can. But, no . . . your journey does not end," said Len.

"Where does it go? I asked.

"It's time for you to make some noise," said Len.

Prominent Points for Chapter Review

- Sometimes there are inconsistencies between conventional medical diagnosis and the indicators. When inconsistencies exist, postpone conclusions and explore all possible explanations.

- The process of intraorgan communication can reveal consistencies between organ imbalances and the conversations sequestered within each one of the body organs or systems.

- When people authentically connect with the deeply seated causes of their illness, their body responds.

CHAPTER TEN

Making Noise

*A*T FIRST, *I was not sure if the remainder of this manuscript and the personal details would be useful to you, the reader. The manuscript could have ended here with the presentation of the clinical research. However, since I told people in order to restore their health, they would have to be rigorous, in all fairness the advice I gave to others must also apply to me. My own life would become a specimen under the microscope of the indicators. As events unfolded over the next several months, my personal journey revealed important information about the nature of healing in general, and therefore, a condensed version has been included.*

I had fun with the challenges of making noise. I published a Web site with examples from the clinical trials and a general overview of the study. As a result, Beth and I received invitations to present and demonstrate our health research at public gatherings. I was excited because I enjoy facilitating group discussions, but most importantly, because I wanted to empower people with the ability to detect the indicators. If they could connect with their perceptual abilities, then they could retrieve information from their own body about their health. Excited as I was, I was also anxious. I expected public demonstration to be the highest hurdle of my career. Oddly enough, live demonstrations turned out to be the easiest of all for me. Whenever I appeared in public, I consistently identified the distressed body organs or systems of complete strangers. My language of indicators had been compiled, and it was simply a matter of using the vocabulary whenever I was called upon to perform.

Since Beth had already learned how to see some of the indicators, we knew that the ability was accessible. I continued to receive invitations for media interviews, but Len and Beth recommended health conferences as a more suitable venue for presenting new ideas and techniques for healing. The opportunity to design presentations was very appealing to me because that meant I could show people how to connect with their own natural abilities of perception and health. Beth and I spent the next several months preparing for a ninety-minute presentation that included live demonstrations at a large health conference. After we compiled the medical data, the bulk of our work revolved around developing a teaching plan that allowed others to learn to detect the indicators. We knew that it would have to be structured differently than Beth's trips to the mall. We also knew that the conference attendees would come from a broad career base, not only health care, so we needed a recipe for stimulating awareness that people from mixed professional backgrounds could equally apply.

Everything was moving forward smoothly . . . but not exactly as I had planned. There were much bigger challenges ahead for me than live demonstrations. During the sixteen-month period of preparation, I attended other complimentary health gatherings to keep my finger on the pulse of emerging alternative practices. While attending one particular health conference, I was invited to join a small group of people for dinner, and I accepted. The morning after, all was not well. I experienced abdominal pain, and my process of elimination was labored and explosive. *A little indigestion,* I thought, which can happen to anyone on occasion. But when my irritation did not alleviate over the next few days, I became concerned. By the time I had returned to my home in Virginia, I was in a great deal of physical discomfort. My symptoms intensified, and I quickly deduced that a parasite from undercooked seafood was most likely the culprit. *No problem*, I thought, and I picked up the phone and called a local physician for treatment.

However, when all my tests for intestinal parasites came back negative, I was perplexed. Other than a broken thumb from playing baseball in the eighth grade, I have lived with optimal health. I asked the physician to explain to me what was happening based on my symptoms, and he recommended that I seek the attention of a medical specialist.

Because of the possibility of test error, I reasoned that I should have the test for parasites repeated by another source. I contacted a well-known laboratory in North Carolina for a second series of tests. When those tests also came back negative, I found myself explaining away the negative test results. *There's always a level of error with conventional tests,* I thought. This could be nothing more than parasites from raw seafood. I was certain that all I needed was a dose of Flagyl (a parasite-eradicating drug), and I knew that any delay in treatment would allow the parasites to spread and multiply throughout my body system. Then it would become a serious situation. But without any evidence from conventional medical tests, a health care provider would not write me a prescription for Flagyl. I became increasingly frustrated with the conventional medical channels. All I wanted was my digestion to return to normal.

I did my homework and found that many conventional parasitic tests can post a negative result even when there truly are parasites present. Without access to prescription medications, I took matters into my own hands. I located a natural formula for eradicating parasites, a nonprescription recipe of black walnut tincture, wormwood, and clove. I followed the eighteen-day directive, but at its conclusion, there was no change to my digestive system. Further research suggested that some parasites can withstand even the mightiest of medical or herbal doses. I repeated the eighteen-day recipe of these three elements with the same conclusion—no change to my digestive discomfort.

I have watched for my own indicators since youth; this happens every day whenever I look in the mirror to brush my teeth or comb my hair. In so doing, I have noticed that my image appears differently in different mirrors. You may notice that the image you see in your own bathroom mirror is not the same image you see in every mirror. Any time I passed a mirror was yet another opportunity to reexamine myself. While I can see indicators for health imbalances that will arrive later in my life, my blueprint says those conditions will not activate for several years, and none of them are related to my digestion. However, with my recent abdominal discomfort, to be extra sure, I examined photographs, videos, and home movies of myself from childhood to present. Nowhere did I see any hint of a digestive indicator.

At this point, I contacted Len and Beth for clarity. We met at the Bethesda office, and I brought my medical test results with me. They reviewed all of my medical data from the different laboratories, and they both agreed with the validity of the tests results: I did not have parasites. I also did not have a digestive indicator, but I experienced symptoms and discomfort from my digestive region. My condition of health was now officially a mystery.

Since conventional medicine was not revealing any cause, I began to investigate other resources. My own knowledge of alternative health practices led me to probiotics; over-the-counter microorganisms that support balance and improve the function of the intestine. I also found countless articles in books, magazines, and stories on the Internet about people who experienced mysterious digestive complaints and symptoms similar to mine and how conventional health practices had failed to offer any explanation, relief, or correction. As soon as they ingested probiotics, their health and vitality were fully restored, almost instantly. The testimonies I read were flattering and convincing, and I could not wait to get my hands on this colonic kryptonite! But after several weeks of popping probiotics like breath mints and drinking black powdered milk shakes that tasted similar to fertilized soil, there was no change to my digestive system.

But I did not stop there. I went on to ingest copious quantities of juniper berries, oil of peppermint, oil of oregano, enzyme supplements, apple cider vinegar pellets, flower essence, milk thistle seed extract, colloidal silver, mastic gum, fiber supplements, magnesium glycinate, deglycyrrhizinated licorice (DGL), and homeopathic carbo vegatabilis.* This is not a complete list, and while people on the Internet reported instant cures from taking any one of these ingredients or a mixture thereof, after several months, my conclusion once again—no change to my digestive discomfort.

Nonetheless, I was determined to reclaim my health, and I continued my search for answers. Surfing the Internet had provided me with many directions to explore, and I followed them all. By now, I was becoming quite knowledgeable about all the digestive imbalances a human being could possibly have. The next phase I went through was a barrage of food sensitivities. The Internet contained unending reports of guilty grocery store allergens. I found myself prowling the supermarket aisles as if I was some kind of dietetic district attorney. According to popular complaints, public enemy number one was lactose, with wheat aiding and abetting. But no food was beyond reproach. I cast aspersions on bean sprouts, lettuce, watermelon, and a variety of other innocent produce.

I persisted along this course even though I was not receiving feedback from my body that my condition was food related. I went through a continual ebb and flow of capricious physiological responses from the foods I ate. One day, I ate wheat and swelled to dirigible proportion. The next day I ate wheat and felt great. Over the weekend, I drank coffee, and my abdomen felt normal. The next eight days, I gurgled as if I was a fish aquarium and could not button my pants. I eliminated dairy from my diet, and nevertheless, whenever I passed the mirror, I saw a float in the Macy's Day parade. After several weeks without dairy products or relief, I missed the enjoyment of cheese and cream. I reasoned that if I was going to be uncomfortable, I may as well eat what I like. I reinstated dairy products

---

*   Always consult with your physician and mental health care provider before making any changes to your diet or adding any dietary supplements.

in my diet, and my abdomen returned to its usual size and felt normal again for a short while. No particular food was coming forward as the culprit, and there was no accurate way to track the effects from any food combination thereof.

The next recommendation I received was to eat only one particular food at a time for thirty days and see how my body responded. In other words, thirty days of eating only rice, and if I experienced normal digestive conditions, then I was to add another food, such as cauliflower. After thirty days of eating only rice and cauliflower, if there was no discomfort, then another food would be added, such as eggplant and so on. The process was to continue until I identified the criminal cuisine. At this rate, it would take several years just to move through the all fruits and vegetables—forget it. My culinary conquests came up empty, and I could not identify any "trigger foods" to explain my digestive condition.*

Beth advised that based on my body's symptoms, a conventional medical assessment by a gastroenterologist, a conventional medical doctor that specializes in the digestive system, would be well advised. I met with a gastroenterologist, but once again, the results were inconclusive, and no treatments were given.

The irony was that I had become someone who came to me for clarity about their mysterious health problems. I could relate to their frustrations as they ran to and fro in the health care delivery system without answers. All I received were directives to schedule more tests. All I heard was that no treatments would be given until tests results confirmed an illness. Since the test results never confirmed anything, no treatments were ever given. My daily activities were greatly affected because of my physical discomfort. I dreaded the arrival of meal times because that meant swelling and discomfort. Most of the time, I felt quarantined in my own home because I needed to stay close to the facilities. My medical bills were mounting into the thousands without any answers or relief, and my abdomen extended to the point that I looked as though I was going to give birth.

Finally, it was time to stop the music! Running from doctor to doctor, from Web site to Web site was only a distraction from taking an honest

---

*   There are people with genuine food allergies and benefit from avoiding certain foods. There are people who genuinely benefit from taking vitamins, natural supplements, and herbal remedies. In my case, none of these therapies were corrective because I do not have food allergies, and my body was not lacking in nutrients.

look at myself. I had gone to the mirror a thousand times before and repeatedly observed the absence of a digestive indicator, and my moisture level was visibly high. But I began to question whether I was the most effective person to read my own blueprint of health. Just as a therapist does not perform therapy on himself or herself, was it possible that I was not able to objectively examine my own indicators?

I had come to a choice point; either I had symptoms without an illness, or if there was an illness present, then I could not detect my own indicators. Even though I can identify indicators and the limiting content in the thought atmosphere of others, it does not mean that my own thought atmosphere is without limiting content. Since I did not see any indicators by looking in the mirror, I now considered that although my body was demonstrating symptoms, perhaps my body was not the source of the imbalance. Perhaps the content of my thought atmosphere was contributing to my digestive imbalance.

I was now in the unique position to test some of the theories that Beth and I had contemplated in the Bethesda office. One of those theories was to create therapies and treatments for the thought atmosphere, but how? Where to begin?

A fundamental premise of many psychological therapies is to identify self-defeating behavioral patterns that we are unaware of in our own lives. We have already talked about blind spots, the area outside of our visual periphery when we operate a motor vehicle. We have also noted that when we become cognizant of our blind spots, we can increase our situational awareness and decrease the risk of collisions on the road of life. As a result of this increase in awareness, our field of perception has a deeper cup to fill than was previously available to us.

I was determined to find answers, and the next resource on my list was the mind-body-spirit connection. I examined the popular trend that you create your own reality—by positive thinking you can change your life. If I define changing my life as healing my digestive system, then all I have to do is think positively in order to heal. It sounds so easy, doesn't it? We all know how to have positive thoughts, so what is the problem here?

I realized there is a big difference between merely thinking positively and ignoring issues versus embracing our life without judgment. While there may be many versions of positive thinking, I do not think that positive thinking means to giggle and think of butterflies, and forget about the patterns of thinking that have shaped our lives and gotten us to where we are, instead it is to regard ourselves in an accepting way.

In addition, the idea that illness is the fault of the person because they "think" in a certain way is also limiting because it revokes our power. There is a significant distinction between taking responsibility for our thought patterns and creating a scenario where we blame ourselves or feel guilty. There is also a significant distinction between having temporary thoughts that are negative versus blaming the world or the people in our lives, thereby getting stuck or hypnotized by that bad feelings so that they rule us, not only in that moment but in every moment of our lives. It is important that people with illness understand that their illness is not their fault. That is not the point. The idea is that each person has the power to live a happy and peaceful life, once they start to identify their dysfunctional thought patterns and how those patterns translate into biological patterns. I went through a long period of changing the kinds of thoughts that I have, thinking all the while that I was changing my thought atmosphere, but the result had no effect on my digestive discomfort.

There must be more going on here than meets the eye because if all that is required to change our lives is to change our thinking, then we would already have a world living in peace. Sadly, these are not the words I would use to describe our world today, which brings us back to our original question, what does it mean to change our thinking? Perhaps before we can pursue that question, we need to pursue this one: when are we actually *thinking?*

Some people might say that thinking is the recurrent narrative in our minds, the voice inside our head that plays the cerebral soundtrack of our lives. For others, thinking is an intellectual process of stringing together ideas, concepts, and abstracts with experience that connect theory to reality. Either one of these models provides an organized cognitive panorama that we could easily interpret to be thinking. Either one can produce ideas that move from the drawing board to the launch pad and, eventually, the surface of the moon. We would be inclined to say that we are actually thinking with these kinds of tangible results. However, when it comes to the personal design of our own lives, the ideas do not seem to move as easily from the drawing board to what we experience every day. What causes this discrepancy to exist? Is it possible that we have been misled to think that we are thinking when we are not? What if what we commonly call thinking is more accurately described as having thoughts?

By no means am I an expert on the cognitive development of the human species. However, with approximately forty years of experience as a human being under my belt, I can make some general comments with authority. By and large, it seems that human beings spend most of their time having thoughts rather than thinking. These two activities are not the same. Each one of us carries large data banks of experiences called memories that we use as reference points to perceive, interpret, and understand our world. As we encounter our daily bread of stimuli and interactions, our memories are coupled to previous interpretations of information, meaning, judgments, bias, values, and decisions from which we derive numerous thought templates. We bring along our past as a frame to understanding the reality we are experiencing in the present. Therefore, the activities of the present moment are often understood, or perhaps misunderstood, by the template filters of the past.

Our thoughts of memories are well catalogued, and we use many of the same templates over and over again as a way of interpreting and understanding our lives today. As long as the stimuli or interactions we encounter are consistent with our past thought templates, our *expectations* of reality and our *experience* of reality equate, and we rarely question how our cognitive processes actually work or what is happening in our lives. When we encounter stimuli or interactions that are *somewhat* consistent with our past thought templates, we have a remedy. We rearrange old memory data, combine templates, and reinterpret what is happening in the current moment in ways that *almost* fit into patterns of thought that were assembled in the past. This near fit makes our experience acceptable to our understanding. When we invent new ideas, concepts, apparatus or creative expressions, it is likely that we are only integrating old thought templates in more complex or sophisticated ways. When new technologies, procedures, products, or strategies emerge, we have been told that these are the products of "thinking" however this may not be the case

Furthermore, if we encounter stimuli or interactions that are widely inconsistent with our old thought templates, we also have a remedy for that—we discount, ignore, or even worse, deny or condemn them. But what if all this mental activity is really a routine of cognitive regurgitation that occasionally produces inspiration but most often produces mediocrity or stagnation?

Since we seldom seem to refresh our thought templates, we often find our lives emerging with recurring themes; our future shapes much like our past. This is why some people find the ideology of changing their thinking very attractive. They are often dissatisfied with the recurring themes in their lives, and if all they have to do is change their mind rather than investigate the origins of those themes, that is a piece of cake. However, for those who pursue changes without investigation by having new arrangements of old thoughts *instead of thinking*, their cognitive landscape operates much the same as the sun deck of the *Titanic*. If each individual deck chair is representative of our thought templates, then what we call changing our thinking, is simply moving the deck chairs around. But no matter how many deck chairs we move, where we move them to, or how many times we move them, our fate or future is inevitably the same—the ship is going down again and again.

Therefore, if we spend most of our time having thoughts rather than actually thinking, could this explain why we do not realize much change in our world today? The nightly television news has the same stories to tell. Perhaps we have not gotten to the root of change because we have not gotten to the root of thinking. In order to truly think, we must consider disembarking from our vessel entirely and leaving the old deck chairs behind.

§ § §

In order to make a departure from my old patterns of thought, I had to find out what they were in the first place. I had to identify the unconscious messages that I project from my own thought atmosphere. I had to see myself from an objective perspective. But I knew that *having thoughts* was not going to allow me to *think* my way out of the bag. I needed to escape my mental routines and reinvent my *thinking*, and that meant a committed environment if I was going to be successful. I pondered a possible reason that people do not have a conscious experience of their thought atmosphere is similar to the experience of when you come home to the smell of dinner cooking. As soon as you walk into your home, your olfactory sense is aroused by the aroma of food. But after a short while, your olfactory sense normalizes to the sensation; you no longer smell the food quite as strongly as you did before or maybe not at all. Since we all stand in the center of our thought atmosphere and have for our entire lives, perhaps it makes sense that we do not notice it; we have normalized to its presence, its aroma, and its content.

These ideas were coming to me while travelling through central Colorado. I was passing through a small town called Glenwood Springs. I had been there before and remembered that the Yampah Springs natural vapor caves (sauna caves) were located in the town next to the Colorado River. I wondered if my thought atmosphere would become palpable to me if I could increase the humidity level around me. If I was going to inspect my own thought atmosphere for answers, then it seemed to be a good idea to make its composition as obvious as possible. The Native Americans had once used the caves for their rituals and cleansings. Perhaps the Native Americans were on to the idea of the thought atmosphere long ago. *Yampah* means "big medicine" to the Ute tribe, and as I turned off the interstate, a dose of big medicine sounded just like what the doctor ordered.

I checked-in at the stately old hotel nearby. As I unpacked my suitcase, I set the intention of my visit to reveal what I could not see, what I could not sense. I descended the narrow passage into the caves with great expectations. The drafts of geothermal heat were intense, and with each step further into the caves, I became increasingly aware of the density of the atmosphere around me. I found an area in the caves that was private and sat on one of the marble benches. I was not the first to enter the caves with the intention to cleanse and heal. As I closed my eyes and freed the tension from my body, I acknowledged those who had sat before me. While the soothing mists played host to my body and thought atmosphere, I knew the stage was set, but if I was going to get to the bottom of my health it was up to me to do so.

Once I settled in between the limestone and the heat, I reaffirmed my intent to be shown any unconscious aspects of me. I sat with my eyes closed, and soon the heated vapors of the cave faded from my awareness. I no longer felt the marble bench beneath me. I was internally transported to the theater of my mind, and my memory matinee was about to begin. Before long, I watched as wave upon wave of imagery flashed by on the screen of my past, a lifetime of moments and possible messages. The vivid days of youth played through, and then my twenties flickered by. Was the message that I had denied myself a career as a professional guitar player to pursue a practical livelihood? Or was it that I wanted to live in Europe and did not seize the opportunity when it came? Countless events streamed by, the moments of joy along with the moments of sorrow, but which one was the important message my body wanted me to recognize? Which one was the *one*? The decade of my thirties flickered by right up until the present moment, and then my memory matinee ended. My awareness was returned to the heated mineral chamber. I felt the weighted support of the marble bench beneath me once more.

My sense of time was distorted. I had no idea how long I had been sitting in the mists of the cave. I was drenched in the moisture of sweat and the atmosphere around me. It was as though the precipitation of my memories had accumulated bodily residue during my review. I was not sure what my body wanted me to see because I had been shown so much. After all this, could I have missed the important point? But as I stared through the heat at the moisture on the living rock, a message filled my mind in a way that I had not expected. The words were short and simple: my body wanted a demonstration of commitment.

I stayed fixed upon the marble bench staring through the mists. *What does that mean?* I thought. Even though I was not sure, I knew it meant that my body was challenging me in some way—right then and right there—but how? I had to honor some kind of commitment before I left the caves, but what? I had approached healing by focusing on the body without success. I had approached healing by focusing on the thought atmosphere without success. Since the two are held in reciprocal bond, I had to find a way to consciously integrate them together—therapeutically. I left the cave with a new approach to healing. The first step of my experimental integration process would begin with the body—by fasting.

In general, our digestive system has not had a break since we were born because of our "three meals a day" schedule. The digestive system operates day and night without rest. Much of our daily metabolic activities are orientated to the tasks of digestion. In the absence of food, the body has a tremendous reservoir of metabolic energy to spend. While the body regularly eliminates toxins from the body system, such eliminations can be highly magnified under fasting conditions.

There are many different ways to fast, and I chose the "maple syrup, lemon juice, and cayenne pepper" fast. The fast lasted twelve days overall, but this included two days of preparation, six days without eating, and four days of slowly reactivating the digestive system at the end of the fast. I received my minerals and electrolytes from the maple syrup and lemon juice. The cayenne pepper acts as a detergent and promotes flushing and cleansing of the digestive tract. This was not a severe fast by any means; some people have gone for more than thirty days. But for my first fast, I felt this would be a stretch and a true demonstration of commitment to my body.*

Many people fear that fasting is intolerable and that the craving for food with each missed meal would compound, causing pain, body weakness, and threaten survival. Believe it or not, my hunger did not intensify beyond what I have already experienced whenever I have skipped a meal on a busy

---

* Always consult with your physician and mental health care provider before making any changes to your diet or altering the quantity or interval of your consumption of food.

day. I had read many fasting reports, and some people described their fasting experience as peaceful, spiritual, and some claimed "divine cosmic reunification." However, I also read reports that said there can be a level of discomfort during a fast. Since the body system is no longer preoccupied with the function of digestion, the toxins that have built up in the entire body system, not only the digestive tract, have the opportunity to release at the cellular level. Subsequently, those toxins move into the stream of the whole body system in order to be eliminated, which can cause physical discomfort. Examples of discomfort include severe nausea and headaches, but it was a chance I was willing to take.

Without eating food, my insides felt normal once more, and for the first time in months, my digestive system was free of bloating, and peace settled within. I reasoned that if a true illness existed, my discomfort and symptoms would have persisted even in the absence of food. However, one side effect surfaced that I had not anticipated or been warned about in any of the literature I had read. My body was poised to release its accumulation of toxins, and for me, that meant burning dry heaves in the middle of the night until sunrise.

Without food in my stomach, I could not vomit; it appeared to be bile and saliva. But I could not make any estimates about its biological content as I held on for the rodeo ride over the porcelain curvature.

The daylight hours were filled with calm, and I could feel the positive effects from purging the night before. The nocturnal hours, however, were occupied with writhing on the floor and cleaving to the toilet while I made my transition from Dr. Jekyll to Mr. Heave. *Better out than in,* I thought with each passing lug. At this point, the fast did not seem as such a bright idea anymore, but I would not allow physiological discomfort to persuade any retreat. My body wanted a demonstration of commitment, so bring it on!

Lying on the bathroom floor on the third night of emesis, I recalled my days in the caves searching for the patterns that generated my digestive imbalance. Although dramatic, I knew this theatrical throw up was not going to heal me. There was more to be revealed, and rolling around on the bathroom floor was only the beginning. It was time to implement phase two of my experimental healing technique. While my body was well into the process of detoxification, I had to interlace the detoxification of my thought atmosphere. Somehow, I needed to connect these late-night episodes with my thought atmosphere, transform purging into power and put an end to this mystery of health.

Without food in my system and having released a considerable amount of pollutants already, I recalled the dense humidity of the air in the caves. I began to feel the raw physiological connection between my body and my thought atmosphere. But I needed to focus while in the middle of these bodily eliminations in order to *clearly* listen to the conversations between my biology and my thought atmosphere. That meant that I would have to unite the awareness of the body and the mind. I reached for my journal that contained my notes from the clinical study and opened to a fresh page. I emptied my mind of all thoughts and handed over the microphone to my body. I wrote questions in my journal and said each word aloud as I wrote. I became the open vessel of receptivity and let my body speak as the words flowed onto the pages in response to my questions.

> What is illness?
> *Illness is not a lesson. It gives us the opportunity to decide about our choices, a source that is given direction.*

> Then how is it useful?
> *It is knowing the source of knowing.*

> Knowing what?
> *The source within is greater than the source without.*

> What does that mean? The source within or without, illness within or without what?
> *Illness is a source that comes without form. Once it moves within, it takes form. It chooses a direction.*

> Can you tell me more?
> *When the source moves within, it changes. It seeks more of the source. If you are not aware of this, then the source it takes is easy. When you are aware, the source it takes loses direction until you identify the source of the source.*

> What does that mean?
> *Illness is a will to source.*

But that doesn't tell me why my digestion has broken down.

Because you don't know the difference!

With those final words, the violent hurls abruptly ended. My stomach released its knot of emptiness, and I slumped against the ceramic node. As my final emanations echoed and faded to silence, exhausted and without a clue, I fell asleep on the bathroom floor.

The above internal dialogue was as confusing and unclear to me as it might be for you. But despite the vague metaphysics in the dialogue process itself, it signified the end to the physical distress I experienced during the fast. The last three days of the fast were filled with peace and serenity.

Prominent Points for Chapter Review

- Unresolved chronic health issues that do not show up in any conventional medical evaluation or do not respond to medical treatment often hold clues to limiting content in your life and thought atmosphere.

- Following these clues will lead you on a powerful path of self-discovery.

- It is not always easy to identify the limiting content that relates to health imbalances. Thinking, by itself, may not reveal the bottom line issue.

- As you peal back the layers of self-discovery, you are likely to be confronted with the duplicity of who you are versus who you *think* you are.

CHAPTER ELEVEN

The Keys on the Dresser

W E LIVE IN a world that tells us to never expose our ignorance. To do so is considered a liability; a sign of personal weakness. Looking good is the unspoken idol of worship in our culture, and the devotion to the *appearance* of "having it all together" thrives in many social strata. Oddly enough, this prevailing approach to life is the unconscious tragedy of the world's stage. People often trade opportunities for growth to wear costumes of composure and remain unaware of the detrimental acts they commit. For some, the price they pay is illness.

The words written in my journal, although cryptically poetic, did not make any sense to me except the final statement. It was now obvious why it was not obvious to me—I was *ignore*-ant. What had I overlooked? I assumed that the unknown message from my body would be clearly evident, but I could not be sure of that any longer. As I read the obscure text in my journal over and over again looking for answers, only more questions arose from my attempts to decipher the words. The fast was over, and I resumed eating, and all my symptoms returned. But the fast had made an important point clear—there was *something* in my life that I had ignored, perhaps consciously.

§ § §

It was time to turn the deepest soil I knew was within me. Again, I would need a committed environment in order to succeed. I headed to the West Coast and enrolled in a three-day intensive program specifically designed to reveal and confront self-defeating patterns of behavior. When I arrived, there were approximately sixty of us in the program; we were all there to examine the unexamined. As I looked around at my fellow seminar goers, indicators of health imbalances were plentiful. However, I was not there to perform health assessments. I decided that I would keep my knowledge of the indicators tucked away because that would have been a distraction from the matter at hand. After all, I was there to restore my own health, or so I thought, but I had no idea what the indicators were about to show me.

On the second day of the program, after completing the morning session of process work, it was time for the group to take a break and have lunch. During the afternoon meal, I sat with a woman in the program who had a reproductive indicator with a loss of moisture pointing to cancer. While we ate, we spoke about many topics, and I was curious if she was aware of what was occurring within her body. She told me how much she had been rewarded by exploring herself through seminars. Our conversation continued, and when she changed topics to tell me about her second pregnancy, she surprised me with her words. While she carried her child in her womb, she was diagnosed with reproductive cancer. Her physicians recommended terminating the pregnancy so she could receive treatment for the cancer; if she delayed treatment and brought the child into the world, her physicians could not promise that she would recover. Her moisture level indicated to me that she had the power to deliver the child and receive treatment for the cancer afterward; termination would have been an unnecessary and tragic loss of her child. She told me that she did not listen to her physician because her inner voice told her to bring the child into the world. She said that she would consider her options after she delivered the baby. I was moved by her courage to listen to her own wisdom as she described the gift of joy the child brings to her life and to her family. She was now addressing the cancer.

We finished lunch and resumed our process work, recycling our negative patterns into positive ones. My abdomen was in knots during a group exercise that combined exerted body movements and verbal catharsis. But no matter the degree of pain or discomfort I experienced, I was not going to stop. I knew the process of self-examination was healthy for me even though it did not feel pleasant at the time. But I was not yet certain what message my body wanted to deliver. I felt as though I was swinging a sledgehammer of wisdom at a haystack of dysfunction looking for a needle of truth. Suddenly, my attention was drawn to the woman I had lunch with, who was on the other side of the room. She was working on recycling one of her own negative patterns but there was something else occurring. Even with the cacophony of sixty people heavily engaged in process all around me, the activities of the room faded from my ears. As I watched this woman, I saw her reproductive cancer losing its hold and slowly dispersing before my eyes! I stood still and witnessed an event I had never seen before. She was effectively negotiating with her cancer.

My mind flooded with words: Is she aware of the affect she is having on her health? Is there a way to medically measure if and how much she is transforming her malignant cell tissue? If I tapped her on the shoulder and told her that the negative pattern she was working on in that moment was addressing the source of her cancer and promoting her healing, would she think I was crazy?

Soon after, we moved on to other points of discussion in the seminar, and she was no longer focused on that particular issue. I continued to watch her, and I noticed that the loosening of the indicator ceased, but the intensity had reduced and her Life Span Moisture Level had increased. The healing power of the indicators became self evident. Indicators can verify when people are addressing the core aspect of illness and disease. By breaking the chains between self-defeating behavioral patterns and the thought atmosphere, illness retreats.

As I continued my own process work of confronting self-defeating behaviors, without anyone to observe me through an indicator lens, I was not sure exactly which patterns were contributing to my digestive upset. There were not any mirrors in the training room, so I could not examine my reflection either. The only other notable event of my weekend was how much digestive discomfort I experienced during the three days. At times, my digestive irritation interfered with my work so greatly that I had to excuse myself from the training room. It was as though my subconscious did not want me to *find out*, and physical discomfort was an effective tactic to deter me from realizing the vital message within. I had definitely stirred up my limiting content, but the cause remained elusive.

Again, I was not going to be distracted from my search for answers. If anything, discomfort gave me the incentive to continue my pursuit. On many occasions, I had told the people who came to see me for sessions that restoring their health would require a certain level of rigor. I knew I would have to live up to my own words in order to succeed, no matter how much resistance I experienced. I had not expected miraculous healing during those three days, but I would settle for no less than a clear directive for my next step.

I was getting close to home, but I had not hit the target yet. Although now my body had become a biological barometer, and whenever my level of discomfort increased as I examined my life, I understood that it meant I was nearer the message behind my digestive imbalance. I often wonder if the purpose of attending the seminar was not about my personal healing but rather to witness the young woman alter her reproductive cancer by dispelling her negative behavioral patterns. I cannot say for sure that she was completely cured of her cancer. However, this confirmed what I had suspected all along. The relationship between the thought atmosphere and the body's biological functions are held in hallowed bond, and I had witnessed this unity in action. I have no way of knowing, no clinical data or proof of the amount of healing this woman caused from her catharsis. I also do not know how medical science would or could have measured this observable event. But I will forever remember the first time I beheld a human being weaken their own cancer in real time by confronting the limiting content of their own life.

§ § §

Even though Beth had advised me to continue working with people one-on-one, I discontinued my private sessions. I was unwilling to do so because I could not unravel the mystery of my own health. As more opportunities to appear in public came forth, I declined. To me, it would be the same as attending a financial planning seminar only to find out that the seminar leader recently filed for bankruptcy. However, Beth and I had already agreed to present at one particular health conference, and the date was drawing near. Cancellation was not an option, and I had to put my personal drama aside and focus on the construction of our presentation.

The teaching skills Beth and I had developed over the sixteen months of working together, while effective for her, were now going to be tested on an audience who was not familiar with my approach to health and indicators. This would be our first time teaching this technique in a formal setting, and we were not sure what to expect.

At the conference, Beth and I presented before an audience of approximately sixty-five people. I demonstrated the accuracy of the technique by identifying the many different health imbalances of three volunteers from the audience. For the first time during a demonstration, I included information gathered from communicating directly with people's body organs. The three people confirmed the relevance of the communication that their body organs revealed as it related to past or current events in their life and their health imbalances. I moved through my demonstrations quickly to get to the purpose of the presentation, teaching others how to access their own perceptual abilities.

Next, I presented a sensory blending technique that the group practiced and then I selected volunteers from the audience who demonstrated rather obvious indicators. Each individual was brought to the front of the room one at a time and stood in full view of the audience. I described the indicators that these volunteers projected and asked the people in the audience to raise their hands if they could perceive the indicators that I described. In a room of sixty-five people, approximately twenty people or one-third of the audience raised their hands.

By the end of our one-and-a-half-hour presentation, the feedback we received confirmed for Beth and me that people can learn to identify indicators on an introductory level in a short period of time. Our next step would be to determine how much variance would occur with individual results and how much time would be required for someone to have a complete command of the indicator vocabulary.

§ § §

After our presentation, Beth and I were collecting our notes and materials when a woman approached and asked if I was available to discuss her health in private. She told me that she already knew the areas of her body that were affected. What she did not know was the cause. I told her that I did not have time since I was leaving very early the next morning. But the real reason was that I was not comfortable offering information while my own health crisis hung in limbo. She continued to speak, and I was moved by her sincerity. The more she spoke, the more I knew she genuinely accepted that she was at the center of her health breakdown. She was not looking for a quick fix. She was fascinated by the information that could be determined by organ communication, and she wanted me to converse with her body in order to accelerate her own discovery process. As polite as she was, she was not going to take no for an answer. Again, she asked me to meet with her. I looked to Beth, and she gave me an odd glance. I turned back to the woman, and I agreed to honor her request.

After quickly confirming her health breakdown via the indicators, we moved into organ dialogue. Within a few moments, her organs told me that her heart had been severed in two pieces many years ago. However, her cardiovascular system was *not* the source of her health imbalance. Her organs told me that the trauma was not from an unreciprocated love interest or thwarted romance. The harm was caused from another kind of love.

This love was so preciously important, so dear to her heart that her life was consumed by the unhappiness from its destruction. The damage was not over either. Her body went on to describe to me the physical appearance of the other people associated with the event, but I could not finish telling her all that her body had to say. She broke down and wept. I waited for her tears to pass, and then she spoke.

Her parents had started a family business when she and her siblings were all very young. They made several sacrifices over the years to develop the business; they wanted a better life for their children. The years of sacrifice paid off, and the business became a huge financial success. Eventually, as her parents aged, the business was passed to the children. The family business was her precious passion, especially because of her parent's lifetime of dedication. But now in the hands of her siblings, she watched in horror as the fruits of her parents sacrifice died on the vine from rivalry. She described in the detail the actions committed by her siblings over competing interests in the family business. Eventually, the rivalry split the family and the business in two, she said, *and* also split her heart in two pieces. She stopped speaking, and once again, the tears flowed.

When she regained her composure, she admitted to having been in therapy over many years. She thought this had been resolved, but based on the intensity of this experience, she was now aware that she had unconsciously continued to carry the suppressed pain. Now, her medical doctors were recommending a surgical procedure to restore her health—organ removal. She had important medical decisions to make. However, she was intent on bringing *genuine* closure to her pain. Happily, she had finally made the connection between her emotional distress and her ailing organs. She thanked me for our time together and left.

As I stood and watched her walked away, I realized that water seeks its own level. Since I was willing to endure the rigors of examining my own life and holding myself responsible, the people who came to me for information were now willing to responsibly examine their own lives for answers. I also understood why Beth gave me the odd glance. Had I refused to meet with her just because *my* own life was not in perfect harmony, the benefits of our meeting would not have been realized. I resumed my sessions with people with the understanding that people can *think* their past conflicts or upsets have been resolved when in fact they have not; the damage is alive and well in the thought atmosphere until true healing occurs.

However, I needed to make some changes to the way I worked with people. I understood the sense of urgency that some people have in getting to the bottom of their health crisis. The way I had structured sessions worked very smoothly and quickly. However, the postsession process was full of delays. Clients had to sign consent forms allowing me to share and discuss our session with their physician, mailing or faxing the forms to their physician, waiting for the possible review of the data by their physician, waiting for return phone calls, and waiting for the client to schedule a follow-up appointment with their physician was taking much too long. Beth and I knew it was time to merge health care delivery with the indicators. We began offering joint sessions with the powerful trinity of conventional medicine, indicator data, and the patient's perspective of feedback. Beth was also able to apply her blended senses with her knowledge of allopathic medicine into a multidimensional therapeutic format.

During one of our joint sessions, we clinically confirmed the client's digestive system as the source of health decay. I applied organ dialogue, and I presented the client with the information that I perceived a large woman holding a stick over the client. The client claimed that no such event ever occurred in her life, and the information could not be accurate. I asserted that the information could be metaphoric and guided the client to search for any possible symbolism or interpretation. Again, we arrived at a point in the session where the client insisted that the information presented could not be relevant. Just then, Beth spoke up from a Gestalt therapist perspective and asked, "Tell me about your childhood with your mother." Within a few sentences, the woman was moved to tears. She explained how her mother ruled with a *verbal* iron fist,which was why the metaphor did not make sense to the client because there was never any physical abuse. As the client went into more details, I watched as her digestive indicator began to alter its appearance—it began to loosen its hold. I turned to Beth to ask her if she could see what I could see. But Beth knew exactly what was happening and finished my sentence for me. It was Beth's turn to watch an indicator transform. Although difficult for the client to accept, her body was communicating that the information was spot on! The trinity of healing had come to fruition. Beth had fully integrated the Visual Assessment Process into her patient practice.

These new developments were crucial to my own health recovery process. Rather than looking for something about myself that I had not seen before, I redirected my self-assessment to find what I had already reviewed and considered inconsequential or resolved a long time ago. It was easy for me to identify the self-defeating content in the thought atmosphere of others, but it was not so easy to identify my own. Perhaps my assessment from the *first* person perspective was not the most effective course for me to take. An egocentric position might actually be obstructing my view. I had to get myself out of the way.

I repositioned the center of my experience to the perimeter and watched the television show of my life from the audience. I perceived all my interactions and situations, from my most significant relationships to the most casual encounters such as standing in line to pay for groceries, as a metaphor for my *entire* life. I refused to accept that there was a hierarchy of experiences; all my experiences were important and of equal value. An observer's role brought forward information I had never seen before. Profoundly, I began to see how others interacted or reacted to my thought atmosphere even though many times, their behaviors were unconscious. I also began to see where my behavioral interactions were automatic or unconscious.

My lifetime experience with the thought atmosphere and the body indicators had allowed me to observe with greater insight. When I was in the presence of certain people, I felt a natural resonance whereas with others, I did not. I also noticed *how* my thought atmosphere interacted with the thought atmospheres of others, whether I was with another person or in groups. The thought atmosphere seemed to have a membrane of intricate small grooves much like the toothed wheel of a gear. When the microconvexities of one's thought atmosphere matches the microconcavities of another's thought atmosphere, both thought atmospheres fit together, the same way that two gears mesh together. However, an extension of complexity exists because the thought atmosphere has a greater dimensionality than a gear—a broad surface area with depth.

However, this information did not completely explain the resonance and attraction. This prospect that my thought atmosphere would only gravitate or bond with those whom I felt camaraderie was not accurate because I also noticed the phenomenon of contra-attraction. For example, if one person's thought atmosphere contains organizing content, or beliefs, that other people will take advantage of them, then people who seek to take advantage of others will be attracted to them. It is the coming together of the opposite poles of two magnets followed by the insertion of a plug into a port. They enable each other. The prescription for facilitating both of their behaviors is filled, and the equation of giving and taking balances on both sides. The way life is expected to be perceived and then subsequently experienced is reinforced by the reality.

I still did not have all the answers, and I began searching other explanatory models for clues to explain the properties of the thought atmosphere. Newton's third law that states for every action, there is an equal and opposite reaction was becoming obvious in my own life. While opportunities to work privately with people increased, resistance from people in my life also increased. Some of my friends opposed my work with Len and Beth. My thought atmosphere was in a "push me, pull you" dynamic of both attraction and repulsion. During a conversation with a friend, I spoke about our recent conference success and how people were able to learn some of the indicator skills. I was surprised when my friend responded negatively and discounted our research. Words escalated, and our conversation became callous when a voice from deep within me spoke, *Why do you allow others to diminish who you are?* Suddenly, I was internally transported as though an ego summons had been served. I had to maintain two conversations at the same time, the external dispute with my friend and the internal inquisition. Both of these conversations required answerability. However, the months of behavioral pattern searching had raised my self-awareness considerably. While the conversation on the outside persisted, I pursued the conversation on the inside and I responded with another question. *No,* I said, *the bigger question to ask is why do I grant people permission to think that they can diminish me?* A tension blossomed in my gut—*illness is not a lesson. It gives us the opportunity to decide about our choices, a source that is given a direction.* My heart began to hammer, adrenaline coursed through my veins, and my mouth went dry. All the symptoms of perceived nervousness came forth, and again the voice from within inquired, *Why do you freely accept such diminishment? Has this become comfortable to you?*

I knew what was happening. *It is knowing the source of knowing.* Instead of being overwhelmed by the activation of nervousness and remaining in a tug-of-war between my body sensations and my intellectual resistance to them—*the source within is greater that the source without*—I realized that the body does not have a built in mechanism for disempowering communication. I had misinterpreted the body's interactive language. These body sensations are actually the body's mechanism for communicating import. Whatever is occurring when these sensations come forth is linked to the thought patterns that disempower one's self. These body sensations are telling us that this particular thought pattern is exactly where we need to go with our awareness. I let go and surrendered and allowed myself to fully accept and experience these body sensations.

Illness is a source that comes without form. Once it moves within, it takes form. It chooses a direction. As my body sensations increased, a greater sense of my thought atmosphere came forth. I could feel its tangible diameter and height and how it actively encompassed the space where I stood. Much like a spider at the center of a web, my thought atmosphere attached my anatomy to tendrils of receptors that extended into the spatial environment around me.

When the source moves within, it changes. It seeks more of the source. If we are not aware of this, then the source it takes is easy. I also knew that what was happening was multidimensional, and I wanted to gather as much perceptual data as I could about the kinetic energies gathering around me. Then I remembered it was similar to the sensations that I perceived when I played little league baseball and how I knew the batter was going to hit the ball. *When we are aware, the source loses direction until we identify the source of the source.* Microlightning was going to strike! *Illness is a will to source.* The distant words from the external conversation grew loud in my ears once more. Somehow, I managed to maintain my participation in the dialogue with my friend; my conscious absence had gone unnoticed. When I returned to the conversation and found myself *insisting* that my friend be kind to me, I suddenly realized the dysfunctional profundity of such a statement—*because you don't know the difference!*

The sperm of perception had penetrated the ovum of awareness, and in that moment, the reclamation of my health was conceived.

§ § §

I understood now why the imagery in the caves offered no comprehensible meaning at the time. The reason no particular action or event held any significance, although that was what I was looking for, was because the message was contextual. I was shown the flavor of my life in *all* situations. It was the opportunity to recognize that I had accepted or allowed a certain level of dishonor from the people I chose to include in my life. Furthermore, I had actually aided and abetted by positioning myself in those relationships so that a disempowering result would occur.

The convexities and concavities of my thought atmosphere were well established. I was unaware of its guiding principles. I had become the fish in water; I did not know I was in water until I had removed myself from the water. In order to smooth the grooves of my thought atmosphere and eliminate the plug ports for limiting content to fit into, I had to first remove the plugs that were already in place. I distanced myself from many of my relationships while I re-examined my personal boundaries. I identified areas where I had set false limits that I believed to be firm. As a result, the crevices began to fill in and smooth the grooves of my thought atmosphere. Once those plug ports were no longer available a new vibration emerged in my thought atmosphere. When I returned to my relationships, the irritation other people experienced in their thought atmosphere because I would not play along with their dysfunctional patterns caused a lot of upset. Some friends settled uneasily, at first, into the new healthy plug ports and they accepted the fact that the friendship roles had shifted. While others simply could not accept my new vibrations and those friendships came to closure.

Two very important distinctions to make here are that relationships are not the only source of biological disharmony and other people or their actions do not cause you to become ill. You must take complete responsibility for your own interpretations, however, you cannot smooth the grooves of your own thought atmosphere if unhealthy connections continue to fill the spaces at the same time.

Shortly thereafter, my abdomen returned to its normal size. I no longer swelled up during or after meals. The months passed, and my abdomen maintained its ordinary size and shape, and the process of elimination was even and steady without ill affect. I could eat whatever I wanted in peace and serenity.

Prominent Points for Chapter Review

- Healing is a process that takes varying degrees of awareness, dedication, and rigor.

- Indicators respond by reducing their intensity and appearance when people intentionally witness the roots of their body organ or system imbalance.

- What was originally perceived as the body's built-in "nervousness" mechanism that disempowered personal communication is in fact a form of resonance.

- Resonance appears in many forms, including body sensations.

- Whenever your body produces these sensations that have previously been identified as "nervousness," it can now be recognized as a physiologic prompt that alerts you to the presence of limiting content in your thought atmosphere.

- Pay attention to all the dimensions of the experience and the situations when your body produces the physiologic prompts. It is a tremendous opportunity for growth and healing.

Practical Application

- Get a partner and sit facing each other in a quiet environment.

- Determine who will be Partner A and Partner B.

- Partner A will go first by looking at Partner B and notice the physical qualities of Partner B (hair and eye color, complexion, and so on). Partner B is to remain silent during this process.

- Next, Partner A will close his or her eyes and notice qualities of Partner B that are not of a physically visible nature. Partner A is seeking to detect any information that is unseen, emotions, personality traits, and so on. Note: Partner A is not attempting to see visions to gather this information. The reason this is conducted with eyes closed is to engage your other senses in order to derive information. Do not be concerned with accuracy; the content is not important at this point. Focus on the different ways of how you can receive other forms of perception.

- Once you have identified the unseen properties of Partner B, open your eyes. Using your sense of sight, look at Partner B and connect your eyesight, what is in your field of view, with the unseen traits you were able to determine when your eyes were closed. Blend these felt perceptions with your visual perceptions.

- Partner A and Partner B switch roles.

CHAPTER TWELVE

Perfect Circle

M Y THOUGHTS WERE far away in the streets and alleys of my past as I sat with my suitcase waiting to board a flight to the UK. This time, I would arrive without any interruption. I recalled the many months since my trip to London had been canceled and how a forgotten phone number buried under a pile of papers revived a universal blueprint of human health. What were once obscure visual descriptions had been compiled and categorized into an identification matrix of health that extends to every man, woman, and child. The body indicators have endured the initial rigors of scientific protocols. The clinical results demonstrate efficacy and reproducibility. Since the body indicators are accessible in a structured learning format, based on our recent conference success, the integration of the body indicators into the health care delivery system seems destined. At the same time, the ability to adjust the senses and perceive the body indicators can be accessed between the bites and chews of a grilled cheese sandwich at a restaurant. The illustrations I provide will accelerate the translation process for anyone who wants to begin their own understanding of the human body's vocabulary of health.

I continued to stare out the window at the Boeing 747, and I watched as the fuel trucks approached. If you had asked me on the first day I met Len and Beth in their office how much I knew about perception and health, I would have said, "Quite a bit." But those estimations were based on the amount of personal experience I had with the indicators before our work began in Bethesda. The evidence of the months behind me and the unfolding cartography of the indicators before me suggest that our human perceptual capacities expand at a rate that I shall forever apprehend. I admit that I know less now than when I began working with Len and Beth, but the mysteries fill me with excitement.

However, to weave new sensory perceptions into the tapestry of the health care delivery system will mean the nonpareil pursuit of uncharted territories. For example, the body indicators could be used to track diseases for which there are no known medical cures or explanation. Lou Gehrig's disease (ALS) is primarily considered a neuromuscular disease by medical science, but the indicators I have seen when I look at people who have Lou Gehrig's disease tell me that other body systems are voicing responsibility for this particular illness. The inclusion of the indicators in medical studies could suggest new avenues of research and direct the attention of scientists to areas of the body that hold untapped information. Since the observation of the indicators is nonintrusive, clinical or otherwise, there is no risk or harm involved compared to the benefits of unlocking the doors to illness and disease. When medical science applies the indicators to create noninvasive diagnostic procedures, the rewards would be invaluable to the health care community and the people they serve (see appendix G).

My observations of people effectively altering their indicators tell me that the body has a natural function for healing, however, these observations also lead me to believe that the course of illness can be clinically reversed once proper indicator procedures are implemented. The relationship between the indicators, the thought atmosphere, and the metabolic life forces of a human being needs to be further explored and understood in order to succeed this reversal. Effective medical treatments combined with patient awareness and disposition would suggest that the synchronized clinical treatment of the *indicators* and *illness* could also prove effective in restoring a patient's health. Therefore timing would play a critical role. Furthermore, the clinical methods required to develop the body indicator treatments could reveal more of the hidden constructs of the mind-heart-body-spirit connection.

Although I maintain that all of the information gathered from a body indicator assessment is valuable, when it comes to invasive growths or body born illness, I consider the Life Span Moisture Level to be the most important information to emerge from the body. This single measurement alone tells me more about a person's health and recovery forecast than all the other indicator information combined and is essential to assembling a whole health picture. "What exactly is Life Span Moisture?" you may be asking. My present understanding of Life Span Moisture is similar to our present understanding of gravity. I can give it a name, I can observe, describe, and measure its effects and results, but to properly define Life Span Moisture and explain the exact nature of its function, at this moment I cannot. I do have some ideas, and much the same as any other discovery throughout history that encountered resistance by the intellectual politics and attitudes of its time, only to be confirmed as true and accurate many years later, I may be limited by the knowledge, technology, academic attitudes or conceptual permission of my day. Therefore, my ideas about the Life Span Moisture remain conjecture at present. I regard the Life Span Moisture Level as the sign of life or the surrender thereof. I expect in the future that medical science will eventually find the correlating physiological mechanism that produces and maintains the Life Span Moisture Level of any human being. However, medical science has yet to know how to pinpoint and measure this kind of biological data. Once found, medical science could create ways to reverse engineer the compositions of longevity and ultimately learn how to fortify this moisture level to the degree that any human being could prevail over any disease. While we continue to wait for those medical discoveries, I am convinced that anyone can restore the loss of their moisture if they are willing to persist in their journey to heal. I stated before that I do not know how to build a clock, but I do know how to tell the time. In order to reveal more of the body's blueprint, I must now make my transition from timekeeper to clockmaker.

I continued to stare through the glass as cargo trucks came and went. People often ask me if I see health imbalances everywhere I go, and the answer is that I see the biological blueprint of every person I meet. There was a time when I focused solely on a person's indicators to ensure reliability during the translation stage. Now, I pay attention to the messages that each body indicator signifies. During my interactions with people, the indicators warn me of the conscious or unconscious invitations to enable their unhealthy patterns of behavior. The observer's role during my interactions has rewarded me with repeated opportunities to strengthen my own self-awareness and personal boundaries. I have also noticed that others may have expectations about my interactions with them, that I will conspire with their self-limiting strategies. Therefore, when I decline the invitation to their unhealthy pattern party or disable their unhealthy behaviors by not participating, I actually create the opportunity for healing. The disappointment people experience creates an irritation in the vibration of their unhealthy patterns of behavior and subsequently their thought atmosphere. It is one way of loosening the limiting content from the thought atmosphere. The gears get jammed, so to speak, when I will not play along. However, I also realize that my momentary interactions with people can only provide the momentary catalyst. In order to restore balance to the thought atmosphere, people must have the wherewithal to notice the sensations associated with releasing limiting content and complete the process of separation. Otherwise, the limiting content will suspend temporarily and then resume its vibrations in the thought atmosphere and continue the destructive directions within the body.

In addition, the recognition of the bonds between the common language of body indicators and the individual patterns of human behavior linked to disease would create new heights of medical and social awareness. Whereby our collective interactions with one another will either promote or diminish the quality of our thought atmosphere. By embracing the metamorphic messages incorporated in the body's dysfunctions, we can identify how we affect our own condition of health from the ways we position ourselves in relationships. This conscious consensual choice to examine and convert free-roaming, self-sabotaging behaviors into opportunities for growth would reduce the occurrence of illness while increasing our collective awareness. Our unconscious interconnectedness to one another could finally emerge as an interactive transformative social dynamic. The activation of this embedded data within our bodies would forever alter the trajectory of human development as a universal species.

For example, if someone has a respiratory illness, then we can bring to their attention the thought patterns they possess that interpret their life's events from a perspective of injustice, the perceptual lens coupled to the respiratory system. During our interactions with them, we can present alternative interpretations of life's events that include compassion and good will rather than injustice. In addition, we recognize that when we impose unjust behaviors upon others, we critically examine our reasons for doing so. Because when we do, we actually catalyze the dramas that perpetuate the destructive patterns of our own health as well as that of a fellow human being.

This is not to be construed as reason to walk on eggshells in our relationships because we fear we might promote illness in others. This is also not to be construed as reason to remain in abusive relationships because our departure might cause others to make certain interpretations that result in their illness. While people may be responsible for the acts they commit toward you, blaming them and holding them hostage will get you nowhere. At the end of the day, all we truly have are the interpretations we make and the responsibility for having made them. We alone hold the keys to our choices.

This is also not be construed as a strategy to commit unhealthy acts against others and then guide them to interpret the acts as otherwise. Do not urinate on someone's head and then tell them it is raining. I am talking about integrity. However, integrity does not come from "what happens" in our lives. True integrity is generated by our response to what happens in our lives.

Therefore, integrity is integral, and here is where the inclusion of indicators during our day-to-day interactions becomes paramount. If we identify that someone has a respiratory indicator but a respiratory illness has not yet manifested in the body tissues, then we can support the *aversion* of illness by interrupting their tendencies to perceive life's events as matters of injustice. Furthermore, I assert that those who perceive their lives from a perspective of injustice are more likely drawn to habits that irritate the tissues of their respiratory system, for example, the habitual abuse of tobacco products. They consciously or unconsciously process or cope with their unjust grievances through this routine behavior. Likewise, for those who perceive life with high performance expectations of self or others, they relieve their anxieties of performance through the habitual abuse of alcohol. They consciously or unconsciously aggravate the tissues of the organ that holds their performance expectations, the liver.

The transformation I speak of is simple but not necessarily easy. By and large, the social changes would be a natural course to us since we are already engaging our patterns of behavior and playing our roles with one another anyway; now, we can do so consciously. This will be the birth of a true paradigm shift, when we intentionally acknowledge this deeply-seated connectivity we all share. Our path of healing will be visible to one another and to ourselves through the changes we make in our lives. Furthermore, the feedback from this interactive social standard would come from the observable changes in our indicators, clinically or incidentally.

Yes, this will require more work on everyone's behalf within our relationships since it is probably easier to remain in our enabling roles and commiserate with the dramas of others rather than oppose the destructive patterns of behavior. But the intrinsic value is reciprocal. As we become aware of our involvement in the patterns of others, we will also recognize how we have taught others to cooperate with our own self-defeating patterns. This expanded awareness would inspire beneficial co-creative, not codependent, relationships as we release the elements that hold the limiting content of our thought atmosphere in place, a thought atmosphere we will inevitably pass on to our children if we do not evolve.

My thoughts overflowed as I stared at the aircraft moving past on the tarmac. Since the language of indicators has linked body organs to messages for our personal examination, the understanding of genetics and heredity could also be expanded. In addition to the genetic traits we receive from our lineage at birth, the body indicators and illnesses that are linked to defeating patterns of behavior have also been programmed into the genetic strands and cell tissues. In essence, the traits of the thought atmospheres of our ancestors are transferred to us through sperm and ovum. When a woman carries a child in her womb, all of the thoughts, emotions, and beliefs that she carries will buoy and bathe her unborn child during pregnancy. Mom is not alone; Dad's sperm brings an equal amount of concentrated colloidal content to the conceptual party. These two gametes merge and mix a broth, saturated with their inherited ancestral momentum, and become embodied in the newly arrived infant. When a female is born, her undeveloped ovaries already contain her lifetime's allotment of ovum. Therefore when a woman gives birth to a daughter, she is simultaneously giving birth to her grandchild's potential ovum. Her ancestral lineage conveys to her unborn *grandchild*, in the biological bouillabaisse of heredity, through the thought patterns connected to body organs and systems; a genetic potpourri of both negative and positive behavioral traits and admonitions. While we are not victims of our lineage or our parents, there are likely to be behavioral tendencies from this intrinsic biological programming. If we remain unconscious to the encoding, then we become automatons of behavior and health imbalances; disease is free to roam our bio-landscapes at will. While some illnesses may appear to come to us through heredity and the genes we receive, it is actually the body's demonstration of the perceptual lenses that are connected to body organs that biologically activate as a result of our behavioral patterns. Remarkably, if we invite the body's messages to come forth and consciously transform destructive behavioral patterns into constructive expressions of our true essence, we could reengineer our lives, our biology, and our lineage. From our casual daily interactions and experiences all the way to the deepest level of our cellular encodings, we could renegotiate the perceptual paradigm of reality and health. If we consciously interrupt the production cycle of genetic strains of illness that are associated with destructive behavioral patterns by releasing those negative behaviors from our thought atmosphere, our progeny would be delivered into this world embodied with the positive healthy loving genetic strands of our ancestry.

As of this writing, by and large, my abdomen has remained at its normal level of health and functionality. I must add though that there are sporadic moments of mild discomfort as a reminder to remain vigilant, and not relax into my old patterns. There are some relationships in my life that I am not sure where their most healthy position is just yet, and I accept that

I am in a process of learning to maintain healthy boundaries. Recognizing the *opportunities for growth* is an essential to any growth cycle. I have been asked after all the intensive seminars I have taken and led over the years why I could not see what was causing my own illness. My answer is twofold. First, if it is perfection you seek, it is a destination that will forever elude you. Living is a continuum, and I know that I will not arrive at a perfected state of being. The only way I can contribute to my growth is to increase my conscious awareness and that fluctuates on a moment-to-moment basis depending on where I place my attention. Second, quite frankly, there were other areas of my life that I felt needed my attention at the time, but I could not get to the root of my body's behavior until I had addressed those blocks in my blind spots.

I have also been asked why my body manifested a mild correctable health imbalance while some people get cancer or other terminal illness. My answer, as of this writing, is that I do not know for sure, but I have some ideas.

What I eventually interpreted from the cryptic writing is that the core of our being, our pure diamond essence, knows the natural harmony of the mind-heart-body-spirit connection. An inner alchemist who mixes and measures the four aspects of being and balances these bonds in healthy accord, this is the source within.

Our thought atmosphere reflects the way we honor those bonds in our day-to-day living. The degree to which we allow or interfere with the natural harmony of these bonds is also reflected in the thought atmosphere. This is the source without. If we dishonor the bonds—through codependent relationships and self-limiting or self-defeating behaviors—then the resonance between our spirit and our thought atmosphere becomes dissonance. Vibrational dissonance interrupts the steady flow between the source within and the source without. If any one of the channels that flow our four aspects of being into our lives is impeded, the inner alchemist does not have the required allotments to balance the bonds of the mind-heart-body-spirit connection. Each one of us has an inherent level of tolerance for impedance that allows our biology to withstand moderate doses of dissonance, and that level varies among individuals. However, as we approach or meet our level of tolerance, the source within or the source without or both, activates. That is why people can have physical symptoms or indicators before any medical test can detect any imbalance. When we exceed our level of tolerance is when our biological landscape becomes fertile for disease.

In my estimation, the reason I had symptoms without any pathology or indicators is the result of years of self-auditing that kept me from exceeding my level of tolerance. Can I clinically prove to you that confronting those whom I allowed to compromise or dishonor my inner source resulted in reclaiming my boundaries and ultimately my health? No, I cannot. Perhaps the timing was coincidental. However, it is compelling to me that my imbalances lasted for a few years, and during that time, I focused on several remedies without success. Once I began restoring balance to my internal and external boundaries, success was achieved. Even if the events of challenging my relationships and the restoration of my health were mutually exclusive and my health was going to return to normal anyway, I will be forever grateful that I followed a path that granted me the wisdom to know the difference between functional and dysfunctional kindness, patience and tolerance. As a result, I have directed my trajectory away from a future shaped by a template of thwarted relationships that was likely to occur. It may very well be that I will work on the quality of my relationships throughout my lifetime, but now I may do so consciously aware and empowered.

Furthermore, the healing I experienced was not limited to second helpings of pasta, double chocolate desserts and intestinal tranquility. Other areas of my life came into resonance as well. By becoming aware of the kinds of thoughts I have, I could trace them to their origins in my past and when they were established. The identification of the motives for having interpreted my life events in those ways defused the charge and I began a new chapter of self-discovery.

Some areas of my life transformed unintentionally. I found that money flowed easily to me. I really did not *need* to work as much as I had before. Work became a choice, and I found myself pursuing personal interests and leisure.

I noticed a shift in the resonance of the people who came into my life. New friendships emerged, and my romantic relationships, which had been challenging for most of my life, became sizzlingly passionate, fulfilling, and fun! I found myself attracted to honest, caring, and loving women who cherished my company.

Another powerful point of perceptual negotiation is to recognize when your body is offering you an opportunity to release limiting content from your thought atmosphere. Whenever you are engaged in conflicts, disputes, or being witnessed by others and you experience the palpable body sensations of what is commonly called being nervous, remember that this experience is actually an opportunity to abandon negativity from your perceptual reality. It is during these expressions of body sensations that the inner alchemist comes forth to voice the feeling of dissonance within that you may not otherwise notice.

Once again, this is very simple but not necessarily easy. The idea of letting go of patterns we have learned to live with, no matter how destructive they may be, can be frightening to many people. Pain and unhappiness can actually become comfortable, but this is truly a mental virus. We have come to accept the thoughts that it is much safer to stand still with pain or unhappiness than to step into an unknown future of gratitude and abundance.

For people who do not have the use of their eyes, the foundation piece of this technique is absent. However, these people can make sensory distinction about their environments that those of us who have the use of our eyes do not notice. I strongly suspect that the people who do not have the use of theirs eyes can perceive textures of consciousness and detect health imbalances in the *sound* of a human voice or what they *feel* while standing in the unseen presence of another human being. Perhaps it is only a matter of making clinical research resources available to them to hone their perceptual skills by providing them with the opportunity to receive confirming medical feedback.

People often ask me, "What is the age of the youngest person you have seen to show an indicator?" I have seen children as young as eight years of age with indicators. People also ask me to explain why some children are born with terminal illness and do not have the opportunity to reconcile their thought atmosphere and health. As of this writing, I do not have a solid explanation. There is so much more of the human being to explore. However, the undimmed senses of a child likely hold many keys to perception and the answers that we have yet to understand.

I was far away in my gaze out the window at the large aircraft. Since my cancelled trip to London, I had made several trips to the Middle East and Asia. I have observed the consistency of indicators in those far-away cultures as well. While there are similarities to the indicators I learned from my Western culture, there are also many variations. I call upon people from all lands to interpret the indicators that are indigenous to their cultures and begin the global transition to social-based healing.

However, one question remains: how do we know when we are actually thinking? I am not sure if there will ever be a single definitive term or categorical explanation that distinguishes having thoughts from thinking;

there are likely to be several indications. As of this writing, one indication of thinking of which I am aware is when you make distinctions about your life that you have not made before. A sign of refreshing your thought templates is when you consciously notice the unnoticed—which allows new forms of cognitive and emotional resonance to emerge in your life.

My thinking was deeply freighted when suddenly an audible "ping" brought my awareness back to the airport in Virginia. Just then, my name was announced over the public address system. I had requested a seat change, and my request had been honored. As I boarded the plane and took my seat, I realized had I gone to London on that day in November 2001, I may have never noticed the piece of paper on my dresser and the opportunity to work with Leonard Wisneski, MD and Beth Renné, MSN, ANP-C would have been missed. The cancellation of that trip, although inconvenient at the time, provided me with the chance to share this perceptual awareness with two open-minded and evolved members of the medical community. I am eternally grateful to them and the kind volunteers who participated in the clinical study. As a result of their willingness to explore another possibility into the mind-heart-body-spirit connection, I was given the opportunity to present a new model of health assessment that has the potential to broaden conventional methods of diagnosis as we know them today.

As I sat looking out the window, I wondered about the synchronicity of it all.

Was this an amazing coincidence? Or perhaps there is a much greater thought atmosphere at work here . . .

Prominent Points for Chapter Review

- The process of weaving new sensory perceptions into the tapestry of the health care delivery system will likely include the pursuit of uncharted territories.

- The body organ indicators have the potential to identify the source of diseases for which there are no known medical cures or explanation.

- Synchronized treatment of the body *indicators* and the body *illness* has the potential to identify new clinical therapeutics.

- The clinical methods required to develop the body indicator/illness treatments might bare the hidden constructs of the mind-heart-body-spirit connection.

- When you shift your role in relationships or you no longer participate in enabling the destructive patterns of others, you are likely to encounter upset and resistance.

- When you encounter upset or resistance from others as you shift into new roles, it often means you are on a healthy track of growth.

- By interrupting the ancestral lineage of self-defeating behaviors and perceptions linked to organ illness (by way of organ indicators), we can decrease the probability of the genetic expression of those traits in not only our own children, but our children's children's children.

- Illness is an opportunity to recognize the dissonance between our body and our thought atmosphere.

- Therapeutic avenues exist to affect changes in each person's individual thought atmosphere and, subsequently, their organ systems.

- *Recognizing* the opportunities for growth is essential to any growth cycle.

- Variations in the indicators exist among divergent cultures.

- Life is a process.

- Living a self-examined life enriches the process and promotes health and well-being.

Practical Application

The next time you drive to work, pretend as though you are going there for the very first time. Drive as though you have never driven through the neighborhoods before, and that you do not know how to get to your place of work. Pay attention to street signs and landmarks, the same as you would if someone had given you directions. Notice how many landmarks or structures you *now notice* that you have never seen before, landmarks and structures that have been in your field of view for years, and you are now actually seeing them for the very first time. *Think* about it . . .

CHAPTER THIRTEEN

Indicators

B Y NOW YOU are comfortable with the notion that people have indicators. If you have practiced the applications at the end of the chapters, then you are familiar with increasing the sensitivities of your everyday perceptions. If you have not yet practiced, spend some time exploring your senses as outlined in the applications. This chapter will support your learning process by examining the details of each one of the indicators and the distinctive ways that you will blend your senses in order to perceive them.

Most indicators are primarily perceived by combining two senses—the sense of sight with the sense of touch. However, there are varying ratios of emphasis on one sense over the other for each of the indicators. In order to simplify the structure of this perceptual process, I have prepared a legend to establish a cartography of these two senses and the indicators of the human body. The legend will: illustrate the indicator, describe the indicator, identify the location on the human body, differentiate indicator topography, simulate kinesthesia, diagram the sensory ratio, suggest perceptual causality, and illustrate the progression of indicator degrees.

Indicator Description

The indicator descriptions represent the physical characteristic of the indicators. Keep in mind that these illustrations serve as a representation but do not exactly replicate the experience of perceiving the indicators

Body Location

The body location designates the area on the body that the indicator is located; this is where you will look with your physical sense of sight.

Indicator Topography

The indicator topography designates the depth of the indicators in relation to the skin. Indicators can be perceived on the skin surface, beneath the skin surface, or both simultaneously. Indicators that are perceived on the skin surface are probably going to be easier to perceive because the optical component is the prevailing sense during detection. Indicators that are perceived beneath the skin surface often require a greater degree of blending of the senses.

Kinesthetic Simulation:

The kinesthetic simulation describes the textural sensation of the indicator. This is the sort of feeling that you need to include with your eye sight during indicator detection. I will use everyday items or surfaces that you are familiar with to simulate the textural characteristics of the indicators. For example if the simulation is "wet clay," then recall the sensations of holding wet clay in your hands. If the simulation is "overexposure to sun," then recall the feelings associated with looking at someone who has been burned by the sun.

It is essential to remember that you are not going to be seeing anything new in your field of vision; you will either notice visual qualities that have always been visible to your eye but you have not paid attention to, or you will experience the feeling qualities of eyesight. While the observance of colors, coronas, or any other uncommon visually perceived qualities apply to other perceptual modalities, those examples are not an aspect of the sensory technique presented herein. However, if you are able to perceive these kinds of uncommon visual perceptions, you may demonstrate natural proclivities to other perceptual modalities. There are resources available today to assist you in developing those modalities (see resource directory).

Sensory Aspect Ratio

The sensory aspect ratio will designate the predominance of each sense that will be blended. The row of numbers on the top and bottom of the diagram measure in percentages. The numbers on the top row relate to the amount of visual perception. The numbers on the bottom row relate to the amount of kinesthetic perception. For example, the diagram below represents that the indicator would be perceived primarily in the visual realm.

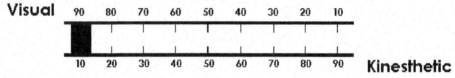

As you move through the sensory blending spectrum, your perception of the indicators will become less visual and more textural. You must bring your kinesthetic sense of touch into your field of view. The diagram below designates a less visual and predominately felt indicator.

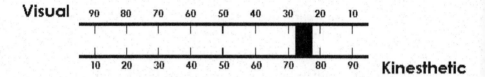

Keep in mind that a less visually based indicator does not mean that you diminish your eye sight in any way or slightly close your eyes. Your eyes will always be fully open and your field of vision in its normal view. The distinction is that you must feel the observable details rather than see them. For some people, blending the senses happens with little or no effort. For others, it takes more time and practice. In the introductory stages of learning to blend the senses, you may consider the combined sensory stimulations nonsensical, convoluted, or an overwhelming amount of stimuli to integrate at once. Do not become concerned with accuracy during the introductory stage. Fine-tuning will come later. Allow yourself to experiment as you adjust to this style of funneling your sensory perception into multiple channels. While blending your senses can present some challenges, it does not require intense concentration. Natural and simple are the keys to this process. Have you ever "tried really hard" to see a beautiful sunset or listen to a piece of music? Probably not, and perceiving the indicators should come with the same level of relaxed effort.

Perceptual Causality:

The legend will suggest possible causality for the particular body organ or system in distress. This causality will not be explained in terms of medical pathology. Instead, it will suggest a relationship between a distressed body organ or system and contextual patterns of perception that are present in the thought atmosphere. The reason I say "possible causality" is because there is no single categorical explanation for all human beings. Therefore, there is no single categorical explanation for why a particular body organ or system breaks down. While I have observed consistencies between perceptual causes and organ dysfunction that suggest a relationship, the ones presented in this legend are not the only possible explanations. These interpretations are not intended to assign people to a preconceived category. While the causalities may seem general, when I work privately with people, I work on a case-by-case basis, and the inclusion of modifiers and intraorgan dialogue will usually home in on the details.

Progression of Degrees:

I have included all of the indicators that I feel can be depicted through illustrations. However there are some indicators and modifiers, such as the Life Span Moisture Level, that I am not sure how to depict through illustrations at this point in my development; I can only show them to you when you are in the presence of someone who has the indicator. Therefore, in order to avoid examples that are misleading or confusing, those indicators and modifiers are not included.

In addition, there are a few body organs or systems that have two different indicators. For example, there are two kinds of breast indicators that I am aware of—one can be illustrated and one cannot. In those instances, I will make a notation that two indicators exist, but only one has been illustrated by placing an asterisk (*) next to the indicator title.

FEMALE INDICATORS

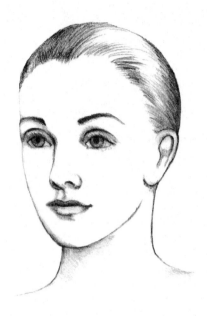

Musculoskeletal
Blood
Blood Glucose
Liver
Digestive
Respiratory
Cardiovascular
Breast *
Thyroid
Neurological
Ears
Spine / Neck

FEMALE MUSCULOSKELETAL INDICATOR

Indicator Description: Reflective surface

Body Location: Face

Body Topography: Skin surface

Kinesthetic Simulation: Shiny, waxy, or polished texture

Sensory Aspect Ratio:

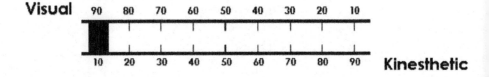

Visual 90 80 70 60 50 40 30 20 10

10 20 30 40 50 60 70 80 90 **Kinesthetic**

Perceptual Causality: Varies

FEMALE MUSCULOSKELETAL INDICATOR

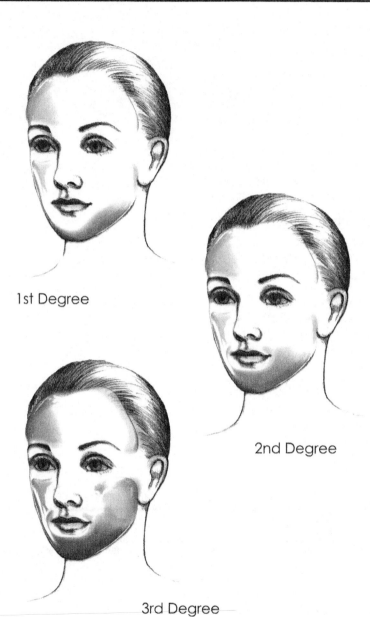

1st Degree

2nd Degree

3rd Degree

FEMALE BLOOD INDICATOR

Description: Personal presence held in skin

Body Location: Face

Body Topography: Skin surface

Kinesthetic Simulation: Overexposure to the sun or wind

Sensory Aspect Ratio:

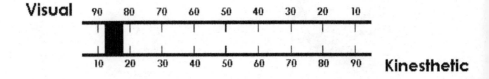

Perceptual Causality: Varies

FEMALE BLOOD INDICATOR

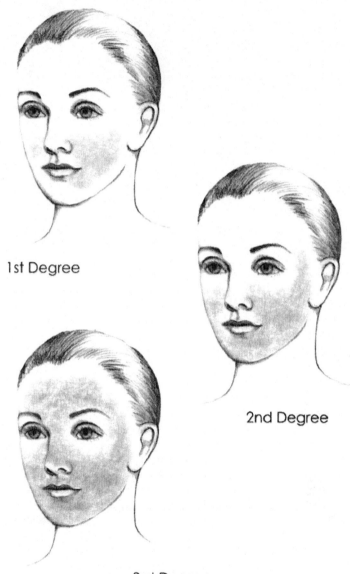

1st Degree

2nd Degree

3rd Degree

FEMALE BLOOD GLUCOSE INDICATOR

Description: Personal presence held in skin

Body Location: Face

Body Topography: Skin surface

Kinesthetic Simulation: Pastel, chalk dust, or powdered sugar

Sensory Aspect Ratio:

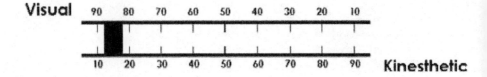

Perceptual Causality: Varies

FEMALE BLOOD GLUCOSE INDICATOR

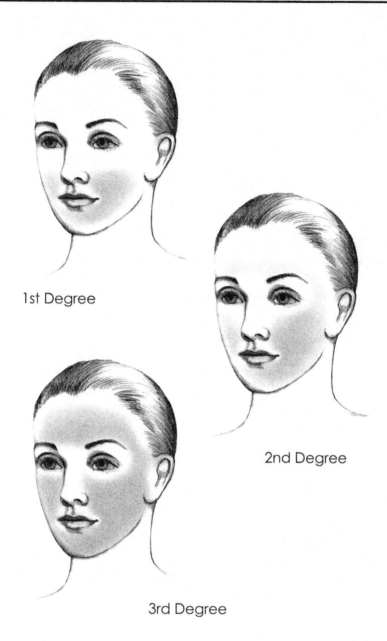

1st Degree

2nd Degree

3rd Degree

FEMALE LIVER INDICATOR

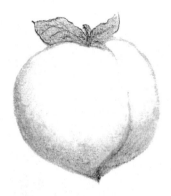

Description: Short hair

Body Location: Face; cheeks, and chin

Body Topography: Skin surface

Kinesthetic Simulation: Texture of peach fuzz. Many women have facial hair, but you must differentiate between hair and peach fuzz

Sensory Aspect Ratio:

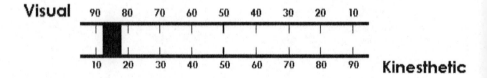

Perceptual Causality: High expectations of self and/or others

FEMALE LIVER INDICATOR

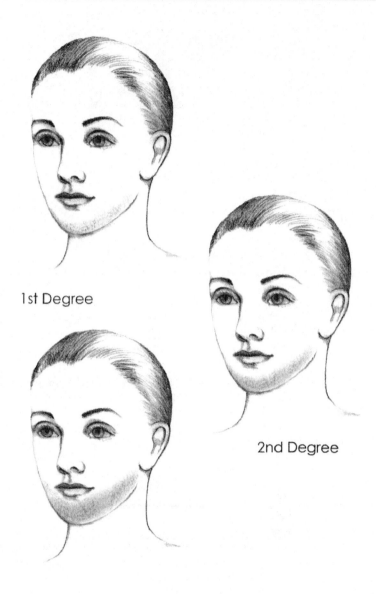

1st Degree

2nd Degree

3rd Degree

FEMALE DIGESTIVE INDICATOR

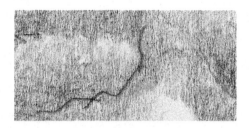

Description: Dark thickness

Body Location: Face and includes the upper torso as degree increases

Body Topography: Skin surface and beneath

Kinesthetic Simulation: Wet clay, mud, or concentrated seaweed

Sensory Aspect Ratio:

Visual

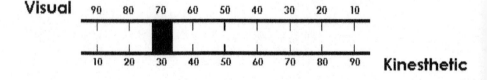

Kinesthetic

Perceptual Causality: The world is perceived as hypocrisy, holding on to the past, restricting the flow of and participation in life, false boundaries

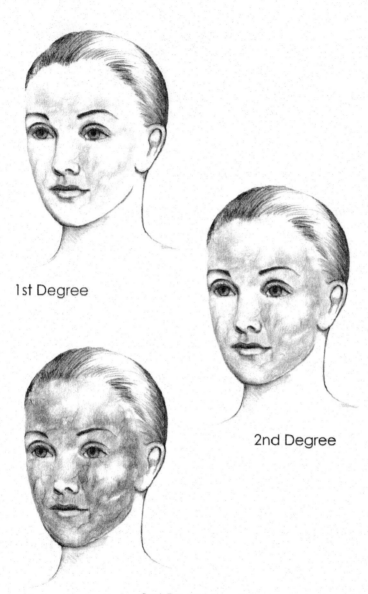

1st Degree

2nd Degree

3rd Degree

FEMALE RESPIRATORY INDICATOR

Description: Granular aridity or ashy

Body Location: Face

Body Topography: Skin surface and beneath

Kinesthetic Simulation: Ashes or fine grain salt and pepper combined

Sensory Aspect Ratio:

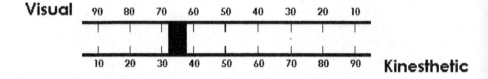

Perceptual Causality: The world is a place of injustice

FEMALE RESPIRATORY INDICATOR

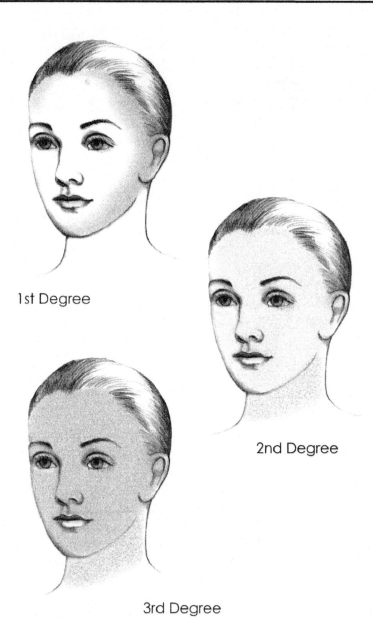

1st Degree

2nd Degree

3rd Degree

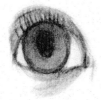 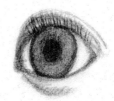

Description: Personal presence is pushing out

Body Location: Face and eyes

Body Topography: Beneath the surface of the skin

Kinesthetic Simulation: Inflation, balloon filling with air or water

Sensory Aspect Ratio:

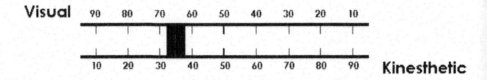

Perceptual Causality: Perceives that relationships need to be controlled, managed, or participated in by pushing people to the perimeter of intimacy

FEMALE CARDIOVASCULAR INDICATOR

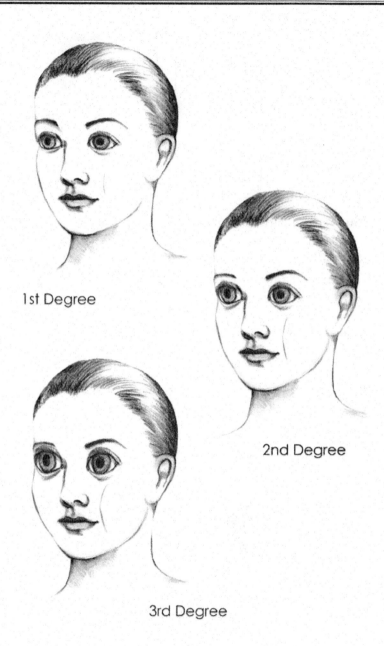

1st Degree

2nd Degree

3rd Degree

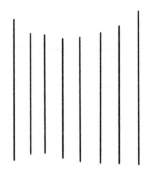

Description: Vertical pattern or grid

Body Location: Face and upper torso as degree increases

Body Topography: Beneath the surface of the skin

Kinesthetic Simulation: Texture of string cheese or piano wire

Sensory Aspect Ratio:

Visual

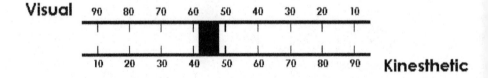

Kinesthetic

Perceptual Causality: Self-critical about the way they have nurtured others or resistance to being nurtured by others

FEMALE BREAST INDICATOR*

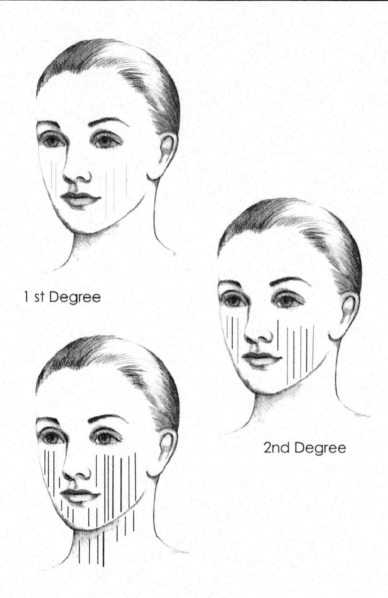

1 st Degree

2nd Degree

3rd Degree

FEMALE THYROID INDICATOR

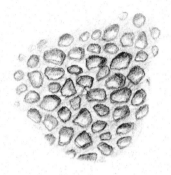

Description: Porous

Body Location: Cheeks of the face

Body Topography: Beneath the surface of the skin

Kinesthetic Simulation: Spongy holes

Sensory Aspect Ratio:

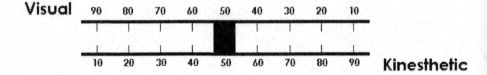

Perceptual Causality: Perceived loss of personal power

FEMALE THYROID INDICATOR

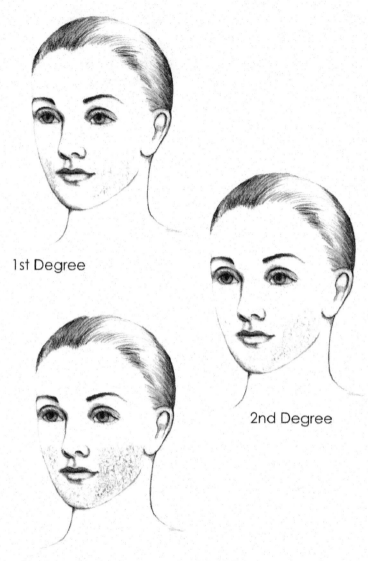

1st Degree

2nd Degree

3rd Degree

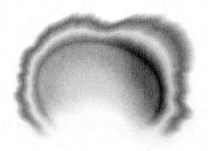

Description: Thinking is heard or a felt sense of busyness or activity

Body Location: Forehead

Body Topography: Beneath the skin surface

Kinesthetic Simulation: Felt pressure behind the forehead, like water held behind a dam. Illustration is not intended to represent light; it depicts force.

Sensory Aspect Ratio:

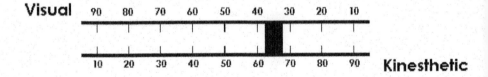

Perceptual Causality: Varies

FEMALE NEUROLOGICAL INDICATOR

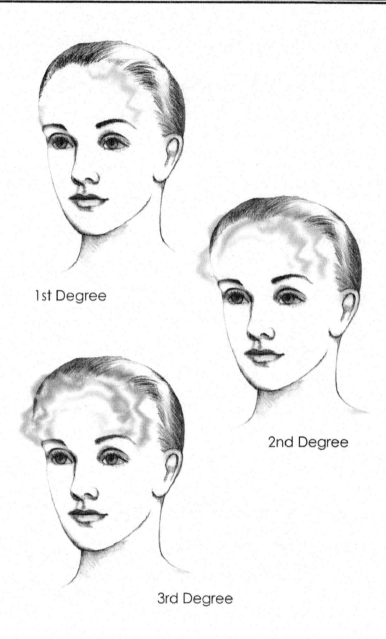

1st Degree

2nd Degree

3rd Degree

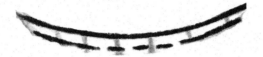

Description: Fenced or corralled

Body Location: Lower teeth and/or jaw

Body Topography: Surface of teeth and beneath

Kinesthetic Simulation: Teeth feel the same as when you look at people who are wearing braces on the teeth. The feeling is there but they do not have braces.

Sensory Aspect Ratio:

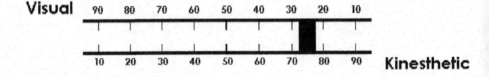

Perceptual Causality: Not willing to examine areas of personal discord

FEMALE EAR INDICATOR

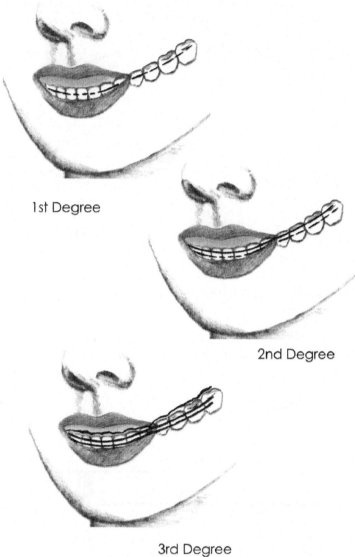

1st Degree

2nd Degree

3rd Degree

FEMALE SPINE AND NECK INDICATOR

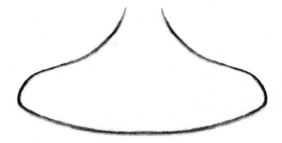

Description: Coat hanger

Body Location: Back of shoulder and neck; perceived from behind

Body Topography: Skin surface and beneath

Kinesthetic Simulation: The frame of a coat hanger

Sensory Aspect Ratio:

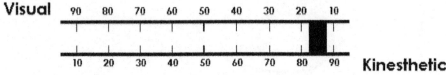

Perceptual Causality: Life without balance

FEMALE SPINE AND NECK INDICATOR

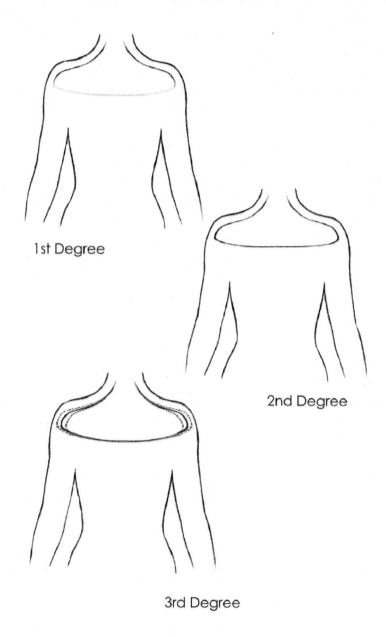

1st Degree

2nd Degree

3rd Degree

MALE INDICATORS

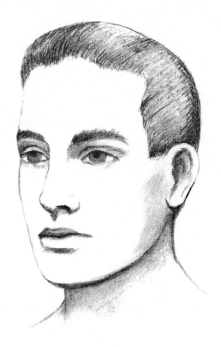

Musculoskeletal
Blood
Blood Glucose
Digestive
Respiratory
Neurological
Ear
Spine / Neck
Cardiovascular*
Genital/Urinary

MALE MUSCULOSKELETAL INDICATOR

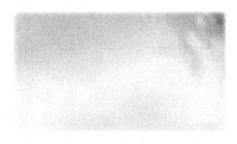

Indicator Description: Reflective surface

Body Location: Face

Body Topography: Skin Surface

Kinesthetic Simulation: Shiny, waxy, or polished texture

Sensory Aspect Ratio:

Visual

90	80	70	60	50	40	30	20	10

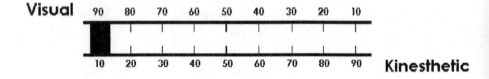

10	20	30	40	50	60	70	80	90

Kinesthetic

Perceptual Causality: Varies

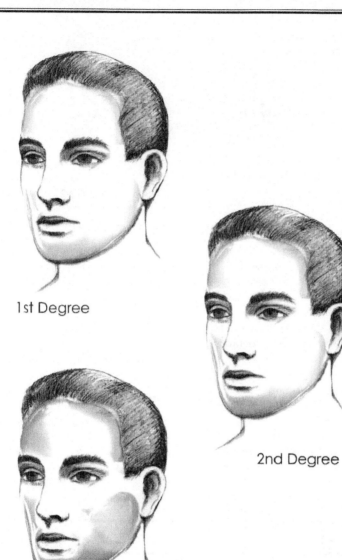

1st Degree

2nd Degree

3rd Degree

MALE BLOOD INDICATOR

Description: Personal presence held in skin

Body Location: Face

Body Topography: Skin surface

Kinesthetic Simulation: Overexposure to the sun or wind

Sensory Aspect Ratio:

Visual

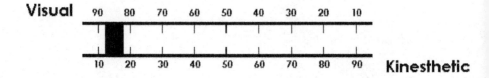

Kinesthetic

Perceptual Causality: Varies

MALE BLOOD INDICATOR

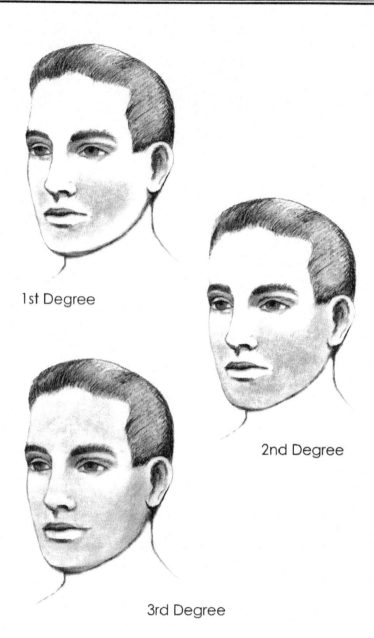

1st Degree

2nd Degree

3rd Degree

MALE BLOOD GLUCOSE INDICATOR

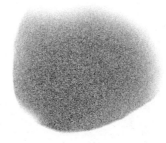

Description: Personal presence held in skin

Body Location: Face

Body Topography: Skin surface

Kinesthetic Simulation: Pastel, chalk dust, powered sugar

Sensory Aspect Ratio:

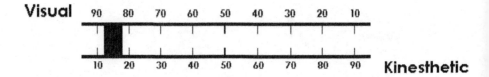

Perceptual Causality: Varies

MALE BLOOD GLUCOSE INDICATOR

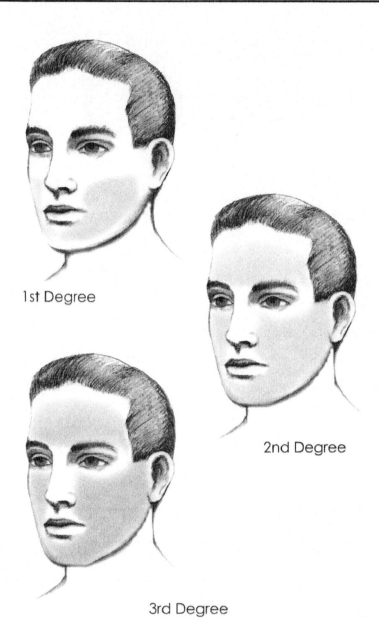

1st Degree

2nd Degree

3rd Degree

MALE DIGESTIVE INDICATOR

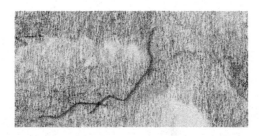

Description: Dark thickness

Body Location: Face and then includes upper torso as degree increases

Body Topography: Skin surface and beneath

Kinesthetic Simulation: Wet clay, mud, or concentrated seaweed

Sensory Aspect Ratio:

Visual

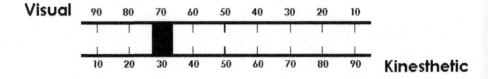

| 90 | 80 | 70 | 60 | 50 | 40 | 30 | 20 | 10 |
| 10 | 20 | 30 | 40 | 50 | 60 | 70 | 80 | 90 |

Kinesthetic

Perceptual Causality: The world is perceived as hypocrisy, holding on to the past, restricting the flow of and participation in life, false boundaries

MALE DIGESTIVE INDICATOR

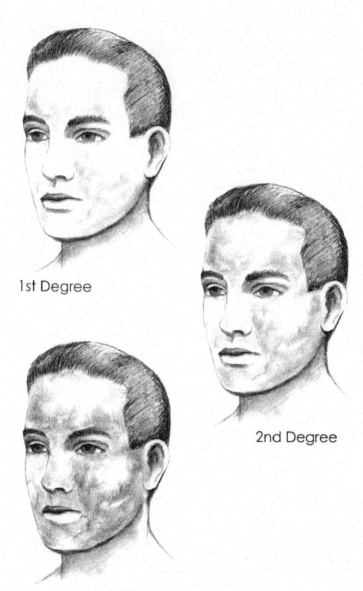

1st Degree

2nd Degree

3rd Degree

MALE RESPIRATORY INDICATOR

Description: Granular aridity or ashy

Body Location: Face

Body Topography: Skin surface and beneath

Kinesthetic Simulation: Ashes or a mixture of fine grain salt and pepper

Sensory Aspect Ratio:

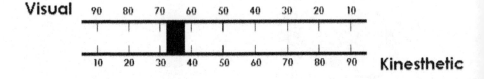

Perceptual Causality: The world is a place of injustice

MALE RESPIRATORY INDICATOR

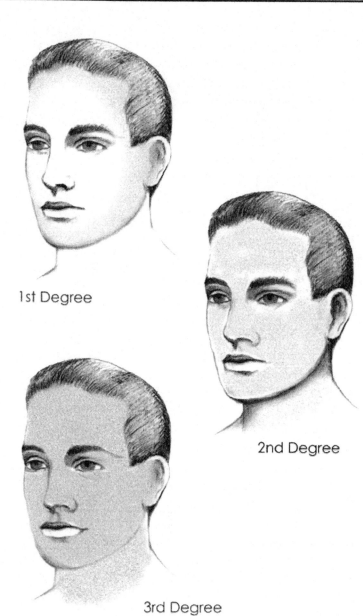

1st Degree

2nd Degree

3rd Degree

MALE NEUROLOGICAL INDICATOR

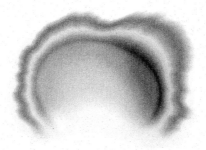

Description: Thinking is heard or a felt sense of busyness or activity

Body Location: Forehead

Body Topography: Beneath the skin surface

Kinesthetic Simulation: Felt pressure behind the forehead, like water held behind a dam. Illustration is not intended to represent light; it depicts force

Sensory Aspect Ratio:

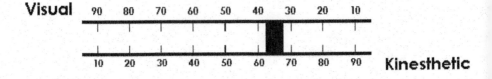

Perceptual Causality: Varies

MALE NEUROLOGICAL INDICATOR

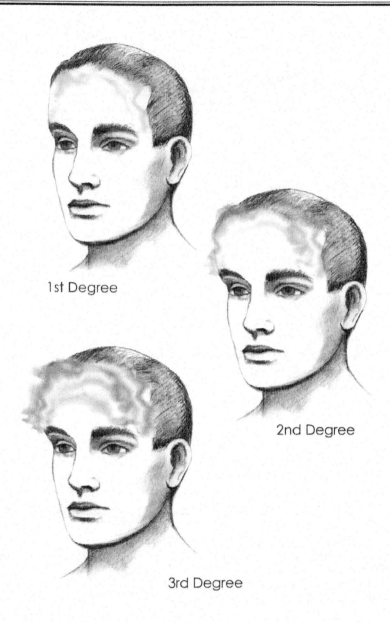

1st Degree

2nd Degree

3rd Degree

MALE EAR INDICATOR

Description: Fenced or corralled

Body Location: Lower teeth and/or jaw

Body Topography: Surface of teeth and beneath

Kinesthetic Simulation: Teeth feel the same as when you look at people who are wearing braces on the teeth. The feeling is there but they do not have braces

Sensory Aspect Ratio:

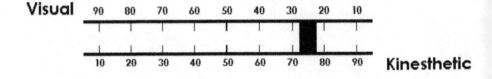

Perceptual Causality: Not willing to examine areas of personal discord

MALE EAR INDICATOR

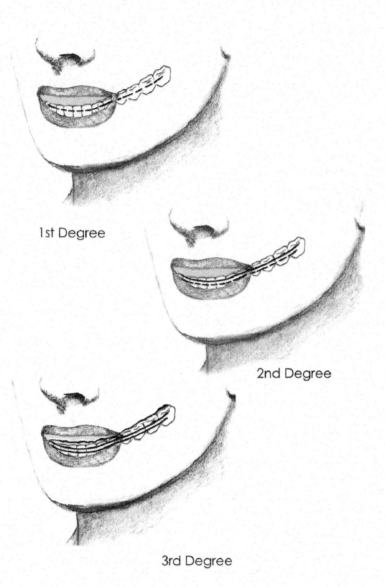

1st Degree

2nd Degree

3rd Degree

MALE SPINE AND NECK INDICATOR

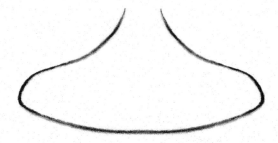

Description: Coat hanger

Body Location: Back of shoulder and neck; perceived from behind

Body Topography: Skin surface and beneath surface

Kinesthetic Simulation: The frame of a coat hanger

Sensory Aspect Ratio:

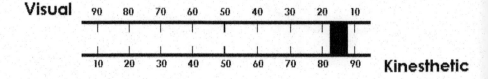

Visual 90 80 70 60 50 40 30 20 10

10 20 30 40 50 60 70 80 90 Kinesthetic

Perceptual Causality: Life perceived without balance

MALE SPINE AND NECK INDICATOR

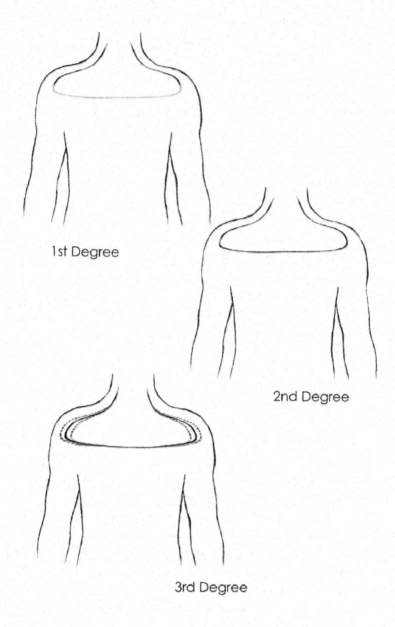

1st Degree

2nd Degree

3rd Degree

MALE CARDIOVASCULAR INDICATOR*

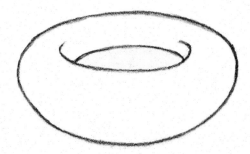

Description: Inflated inner tube or rings

Body Location: Around the area of the chest, below the armpit

Body Topography: Skin surface and beneath. Sometimes extends beyond the skin surface

Kinesthetic Simulation: Inner tube around the chest

Sensory Aspect Ratio:

Visual

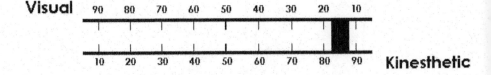

Kinesthetic

Perceptual Causality: Fortress around the heart, keeps people/relationships at arm's length

MALE CARDIOVASCULAR INDICATOR*

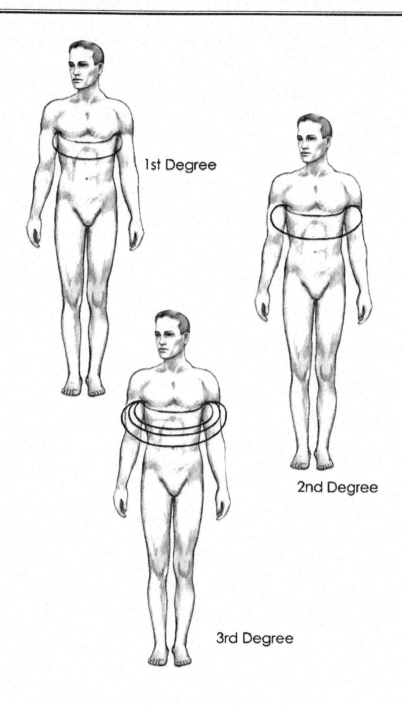

1st Degree

2nd Degree

3rd Degree

MALE GENITAL / URINARY INDICATOR

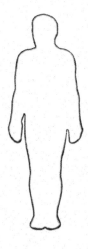

Description: Hollow frame

Body Location: Body periphery

Body Topography: Skin surface and extends beyond

Kinesthetic Simulation: Frame without a picture

Sensory Aspect Ratio:

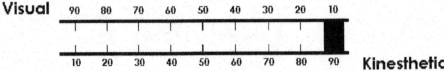

Perceptual Causality: The world is not a safe place

MALE GENITAL / URINARY INDICATOR

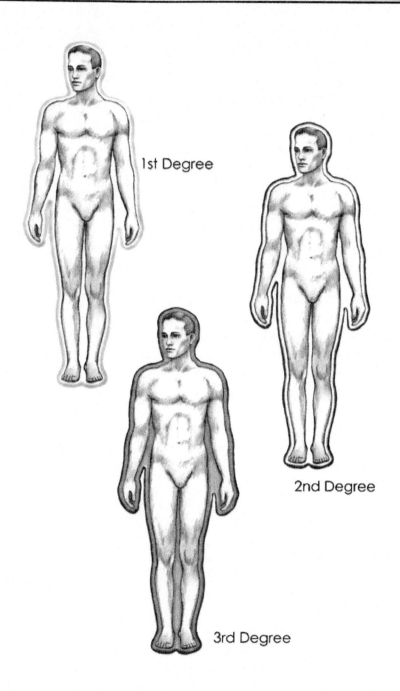

1st Degree

2nd Degree

3rd Degree

APPENDIX A

_____ Leonard Wisneski, MD
_____ Beth Renne' ANP-C

NEW PATIENT PROGRESS NOTE

PATIENT NAME: _____

Vital Signs: Height _____ Weight _____

B/P _____ Pulse _____

SUBJECTIVE	
HPI	
Onset	
Location	
Duration	
Characteristics	
Aggravating factors	
Relieving factors	
(Rx, conventional alternative treatment, other)	
Related symptoms, Health problems, Complications	
Related life issues	
Emotional	
Areas of stress	
Psychosocial	
Dysfunctional issues	
Social	
Family	
Job	
Financial	
OBJECTIVE	
HEENT	
Respiratory	
Cardiac	
GI	
GU	
Skin	
Extremities	
Neuro	
ASSESSMENT	
HEALING PATH	
Lab/other tests	
Acupuncture	
Body work/chiropractic	
Soft tissue therapies	
Counseling	
Nutrition	
Medications	
Rx	
Nutriceuticals	
Herbs	
Supplements	
Reading	
Classes	
Yoga	
Tai chi	
Qi gong	
FOLLOW–UP	

_____
Provider's Signature   Date

APPENDIX B

Intuitive Health Assessment Form

Intuitive perception is a way of receiving information using capabilities beyond the process of logical reasoning and the use of our usual five sensory systems. It is plausible, that this type of perception has utility in the evaluation and treatment of medical conditions.

John Kortum is an *intuitive health counselor*. Since his early childhood, he has been aware of his ability to perceive information intuitively. He has recently become interested in exploring its use in medicine. To this end, John has developed a specific method and accompanying vocabulary that organizes this information into a tool that allows access to it in a clear, concise manner.

In an effort to explore this previously untapped well of potential information, we have designed an exploratory pilot study that compares intuitively based medical information with medical information collected using the traditional medical framework.

Patients who voluntarily elect to become partners in this effort will undergo two medical examinations. The first will be a traditional physical exam, including history, physical and routine laboratory studies. The second will be an *intuitive* assessment in which intuitively based information regarding a person's health will be received by observation of personal presence and energetic field. A short period of observation is required (one to three minutes) in order to assess major body systems (digestive, cardiovascular, endocrine, reproductive, etc.) It is necessary for the examiner (John) not to know your medical history. During your time together, you may feel free to speak or you can remain silent, whichever you prefer. The examiner will be available to answer any questions that you may have about the information he receives. The results of the intuitive assessment will not be considered part of your formal medical records, however, the information collected may prove useful as a basis for further conventional medical evaluation, if you so choose.

Each of the assessments will be performed separately. After all the information is collected, the results will be compared with particular attention to details that appear consistently in both the traditional medical and the intuitive realm.

All records will be kept confidential. If all or part of them is published as part of the study, confidentiality will be upheld.

The potential use of intuitive assessments as a tool for healing represents a giant step forward in the theory and practice of modern medicine. As a participant in this study, you can be a partner in uncovering some of the deepest secrets that lie within the undiscovered realm of human potential.

I, _____, voluntarily, knowingly, and willingly give my consent to receive an Intuitive Health Assessment as outlined above. I have been adequately informed, and any questions I have asked have been satisfactorily answered. I acknowledge that I am seeking this form of assessment solely for the purpose of understanding my own health and wellness. I also understand that the results of this assessment may be used as part of a research study where complete confidentiality will be upheld. I am aware that I may withdraw this consent at any time.

APPENDIX C

Indicator Health Assessment Form

Patient Name: _____ **Age:** _____ **Date:** _____

Review of Systems	Body Indicators		YES	NO
1 General _____	Is Ash present?	1		
2 HEENT _____	Is Wired or Framed present?	2		
3 Respiratory _____	Is Dirty present	3		
4 Cardiac _____	Is Curvature present?	4		
5 GI _____	Dark/Thickness present?	5		
6 GU Men _____	Hollow Frame present?	6		
7 GU Women _____	Moisture present?	7		
7a If Yes>	Is Moisture Dormancy present?	7a		
8 Blood _____	Is presence held in skin?	8		
8a If Yes>	Is Blood Carrier or Illness Specific?	8a		
8b If No>	Is presence held in skin "pastel"?	8b		
9 Neurological _____	Is Thinking heard?	9		
9a Spinal/neck If No>	Is Coat Hanger Present?	9a		
10 Breast _____	Is Strained present?	10		
10a If No>	Is Bird present?	10a		
11 Glands _____	Is Sponge/Holes present?	11		
12 Muscular/Skeletal _____	Is presence waxy?	12		
13 Eyes _____	Is illumination present?	13		

Outliers
Is presence Unusual/Extreme?

	YES	NO

Comments:

_____
_____
_____
_____

APPENDIX D

Study Protocol

Each of the patients met with John in a medical office examination room.

John met the patients on the day of testing and only at the moment when the testing was performed.

John was given no past or current health, heredity or lifestyle information relating to the patient.

John would sit within four to six feet of the patient and observe their presence.

The patient and John were the only people in the room.

The patients selected were not demonstrating any outward signs of health abnormalities during the visual assessment. For example, no one used crutches; no one wore casts or bandages; no one had open wounds; no one had visible surgery marks, scars, or stitches; no one had audible symptoms such as coughing, sneezing or sinus congestion; and so on.

The patients did not communicate any symptoms or complaints, written or oral.

Each patient was also evaluated using the conventional medical model by Beth Renné, ANP-C.

APPENDIX E

Indicator Health Assessment Form   MALE

Patient Name _____   Age: ____   Date: ___

Review of Systems	Body Indicators		YES	NO		Degree 1 2 3			Notes

Review of Systems	Body Indicators			
1 General	Is Dirty or Ashy?	1		
2 Ear	Is Jaw Wired or Framed?	2		
3 Eyes	Is Dark Thickness present?	3		
4 Respiratory	Is Dirty present?	4		
4a If Yes>	Is Shield Present?	4a		
5 Cardiac	Is Curvature present?	5		
6 GI Large/Colon	Dark/Thickness present?	6		
6a Small/Stomach	Mild Dark Thickness?	6a		
6b GB, P. S.	Porous Mild Dark Thickness?	6b		
6c Liver	Spotted present?	6c		
7 GU Male	Hollow Frame present?	7		
7a If No>	Moisture present?	7a		
8 Blood	Is Presence held in skin?	8		
8a If Yes>	Is Blood Carrier or Illness Specific?	8a	BC	IS
8b If Yes>	Is Presence held in skin "pastel"?	8b		
8c If No>	Is Strained present?	8c		
8d If No>	Holes/Sponge present?	8d		
9 Neurological	Is Thinking heard?	9		
10 Spinal/neck	Is Coat Hanger Present?	10		
11 Throat/Esophagus	Is Stork/Bird Present	11		
12 If Yes>	Dirty/Ashy?	12		
13 Muscular/Skeletal	Is Presence Waxy?	13		
14 Thyroid	Holes/Sponge present?	14		

Outliers

			YES	NO
15 Evasive/disguised	Is presence Unusual/Extreme?	15		

Modifiers

16 Unique Indicators		16	

17 Respond to queries?		17	

18 Intra Organ Communcation   ____ %
19 Life Span Moisture Level   ____ %

Comments:
_____
_____
_____
_____
_____

APPENDIX F

Indicator Assessment Form FEMALE

Patient Name: _____ Age: ____ Date: ____

Review of Systems	Body Indicators		YES	NO		Degree 1	2	3	Notes
1 General	Is Dirty or Ashy?	1							____
2 Ear	Is Jaw Wired or Framed?	2							____
3 Eyes	Is Dark Thickness Present?	3							____
4 Respiratory	Is Dirty present?	4							____
4a If Yes>	Is shield Present?	4a							____
5 Cardiac	Is presence pushing out?	5							____
6 GI Large/Colon	Heavy Dark/Thickness present?	6							____
6a Small/stomach	Mild Dark/ Thickness present?	6a							____
6b P.S.GB.	Porous Mild Dark Thickness?	6b							____
6c Liver	Peach fuzz present?	6c							____
7 GU Female	Glossy moisture present?	7							____
7a If Yes>	Is Moisture Dormancy present?	7a							____
8 Blood	Is Presence held in skin?	8							____
8a If Yes>	Is Blood Carrier or Illness Specific?	8a	BC	IS					____
8b If No>	Is Presence held in skin "pastel"?	8b							____
9 Neurological	Is Thinking Heard?	9							____
10 Spinal / Neck	Is Coat Hanger Present?	10							____
11 Breast	Is Strained present?	11							____
11a If No>	Is Bird present?	11a							____
12 Thyroid	Holes/Sponge present?	12							____
13 Muscular/Skeletal	Is Presence Waxy?	13							____
14 Throat/Esophagus	Is Stork Present?	14							____

Outliers

			YES	NO					
15 Evasive/Disguised	Is energy Unusual/Extreme?	15							

Modifiers

16 Unique Indicators		16							

17 Respond to queries?		17			

18 Intra Organ Communcation			%
19 Life Span Moisture Level			%

Comments:

_____
_____
_____
_____
_____

APPENDIX G

Test Study

TERMS

Conventional medical assessment tools/findings: Represent the traditional medical model as it is practiced today, and includes a medical history, physical examination, and laboratory studies.

The Kortum Technique assessment tool/findings: Represent evaluation through a *sensory pathway.* This form of perception is *intuitive* and the information that is received or known through this process exists beyond the process of logical reasoning and the use of our ordinary five sensory system. The assessment is performed *visually* by direct observation of personal presence and energetic field.

Indicators: Visible symbology that identifies the body system or organ.

ABSTRACT

The study was performed in order to compare and evaluate the consistencies between the results of health assessments performed using the conventional medical model and the use of a specific sensory observation technique (the Kortum Technique). The sensory observation technique identified the conventional medical diagnoses with numeric accuracy of 0.9347 or about 90%. Additional research is needed in order to demonstrate statistical reliability and validity.

INTRODUCTION

This study is designed to investigate whether there are consistencies between the results of health assessments performed using the conventional medical model and the use of a sensory observation technique. If substantiated by the scientific process, the technique will portend tremendous potential in the medical field, including but not limited to the development of new health assessment procedures, renewed consideration of the nature of illness and disease, and the identification of heretofore unknown factors in the ways that illness and disease manifest in patients.

METHODS

Subject Recruitment

Subjects were recruited through word of mouth as well as from a patient population pool connected to a small internal medicine practice in Bethesda, Maryland.

Data Collection

Each participant was mailed a packet containing an introductory letter, informed consent forms, and a patient intake form. They were instructed to read all the materials and fill out the intake form.

Each subject was then given an appointment for the in-person assessment procedure. During their office visit, the research protocol was reviewed and the informed consent was signed and witnessed. Each of the two assessment tools was employed. Data was collected and recorded for each subject.

Protocol

Each of the subjects met with the examiner in a medical office examination room. The examiner had not met the subjects prior to the day of testing and was given no past or current health history about the subject. He sat within four to six feet of the subject and observed their presence. Using the observation technique, the level of performance accuracy was determined by how many times the observation technique identified a body organ or system as having an abnormality when there was a correlating confirmed conventional medical diagnosis.

Limitations

The Kortum Technique identified health imbalances in patients that could not be included in the study results for the following reasons:

- Patient subjects complained of discomfort and symptoms, but the conventional medical assessment could not offer a diagnosis.

- Some health imbalances that were identified by the observation technique at the time of testing were not supported by a conventional medical diagnosis until after the research period was concluded.

DISCUSSION

The exploratory nature of the work was intended primarily to uncover potential avenues for future study and not to prove the validity or reliability of the observation technique. A formal statistical study and analysis at a later date will be required in order to determine if the technique will meet the rigors of the scientific process. The results of the pilot study indicate that the two assessment tools appear to disclose fairly consistent information.

IMPLICATIONS

The Kortum Technique exceeds our current understanding of when illness or disease is actually detectable in the human body.

Many conversations took place during the course of the study. As a result, we came up with a number of questions that relate to the different types of assessment and to the general importance of this work.

Our first and most important questions were:

- Where do we go from here?
- Do we feel confident enough to state that these assessment tools, based on our pilot study data, have enough of a promise of reliability to warrant further research?
- Do we have enough information to construct a clear hypothesis?
- What might that hypothesis be?

Further questions that relate to the nature of the Kortum Technique were:

1. How is the Kortum Technique properly defined?
2. How does the Kortum Technique actually work? What is the *organ* that does the perceiving? Does it have a structure?

3. What differentiates the observation technique and medical intuitive perception?
4. What is its potential for future study?
5. How can this mode of evaluation be used to empower people on their journey towards health and wholeness?

More specifically . . .

1. Can this type of assessment be used to recommend conventional or alternative medical treatment?
2. Can this type of assessment be used to evaluate energetic alterations that could support or guide treatment of a transpersonal nature (soul work)?
3. Is there a difference in the treatment outcomes using this process between subjects who understand and believe in the energetic universe versus those who do not?
4. Can this process be used to evaluate the effectiveness of present treatment modalities based on normalization of previously noted changes in the energetic field?

Even more specifically . . .

1. We have identified that there is some aspect of inter- and intra-body and inter- and intra-organ communication. How can that be used as a basis for evaluating health and/or spiritual issues?
2. Does everyone's body speak the same language as reflected through the visual indicators in this assessment tool?
   (People's bodies seem to send out the same indicators in the presence of similar disease processes—diabetes indicators, thyroid indicators, blood indicators, and even, we suspect, indicators related to traditional Chinese medical diagnoses.)
3. What are the conversations the body is having and why?
4. Does the development of a disease happen regardless of what we do if we need a life lesson?

We identified the following items as steps to further the scientific exploration of this topic:

1. Design a scientific study that tests for validity, reliability, sensitivity, and specificity.
2. Determine if the Kortum Technique is universally teachable.
3. Create a therapeutic modality using this process and test it to see if it is useful in connecting people to their own authentic power and healing, using integrative medicine as a basis.

CONCLUSION

The work introduced has brought forth many questions, possibilities, potentials and opportunities for future study. Its implications regarding the way we, as health care providers assess, evaluate and treat health and disease are far reaching. They expand the basis not only of our knowledge structure but also of our methods of perceiving health, disease, and its relationship to the human condition. As we move to address these questions, we forge the future of medicine with open hearts, minds, and spirits and dedicate ourselves to supporting the evolution of this *new medicine* that integrates and embraces all of the depth and complexity—that is, the human organism.

FREQUENTLY ASKED QUESTIONS

Why would I choose to include the Kortum Technique in my healing discovery process?

If your health imbalance has been correctly identified and you are experiencing progress, congratulations, you are moving toward wholeness of health. If you are experiencing confusion about your health or your imbalances persist without resolution, then the Kortum Technique is an excellent tool to begin revealing the sources of your health imbalance.

How do I know if the Kortum Technique is for me?

In addition to the Kortum Technique being applied when conventional methods are not able to identify the cause, the technique also presents information about the status of a past or present imbalance as well as offering indications of a possible future health imbalance. Some people are simply interested in a general indicator check-up.

What happens during the Visual Assessment Process?

The Kortum Technique is conducted in a conversational setting and has three essential components. During the first component, the technique is used to survey the indicators that might be present. Information can also be surveyed about the level of activity for those indicators. Further discussion will allow you the opportunity to provide feedback about what you already know about your health compared to the indicator evaluation.

The second component is dedicated to revealing what your body wants to communicate. The organs can describe past events in your life but most likely will speak in metaphoric terms or symbols that relate to any history that might motivate the health imbalance. Sometimes, the organs are reluctant or unwilling to communicate, which often parallels a situation where the client is having difficulty acknowledging or examining their own limiting content.

The third component will be your opportunity to consider what has been revealed in the session and how you can use this information to best support your recovery of health and vitality.

How does the Kortum Technique actually work?

The human body has a symbolic language to indicate health imbalances within the different organ and systems. When the imbalance reaches a certain threshold, it activates this symbolic language and becomes visible and accessible through the Kortum Technique.

Will the Kortum Technique heal or cure me?

People have varying rates of recovering from any health imbalance. The Kortum Technique is a discovery process and can reveal much about the relationship you have with your body. For some people, core aspects of illness and disease become illuminated during a session. For others, they recognize that their path to healing may require certain therapies, and it is time to pursue those therapies through appropriate channels. Depending on your case, it is likely that you will continue to work with your health care provider for a period of time until you achieve wellness. The Kortum Technique is not a quick fix, the Kortum Technique is not a substitution for medical treatment, the Kortum Technique does not diagnose, treat, cure, or alleviate an illness in any way, the Kortum Technique is also not a way to supersede the unconscious messages that your body is bringing forward. A session can be a powerful first step in your own amazing journey of returning to health and vitality.

Will the Kortum Technique render scientifically detailed data and diagnose my health condition?

The symbolic language of your body will designate if a certain organ or system is demonstrating an indicator and also give details about the intensity. Scientific or medically diagnostic questions—such as, "What is the mercury or glucose level content of my blood?" or "Do I have cancer?"—are outside the scope of a session and are questions for you to pursue with your health care provider. A session will focus solely on the unconscious patterns of illness and how to bring these patterns forward to be useful in your healing process.

ONLINE RESOURCE DIRECTORY

http://www.JohnKortum.com

The Hoffman Institute
http://www.hoffmaninstitute.org

The Monroe Institute
http://www.monroeinstitute.org

CPSIA information can be obtained at www.ICGtesting.com
Printed in the USA
BVOW08s1336081015

421354BV00003B/280/P